between
patient
and
health worker

between patient and health worker

THELMA LEE DORROH
Associate Professor
Department of Community Health and Medical Practice
School of Medicine
University of Missouri

McGraw-Hill Book Company
A Blakiston Publication
New York   St. Louis   San Francisco   Düsseldorf   Johannesburg
Kuala Lumpur   London   Mexico   Montreal   New Delhi
Panama   Paris   São Paulo   Singapore   Sydney   Tokyo   Toronto

to WILLIAM D. BRYANT

But for him this book would never have been written

This book was set in Optima by Black Dot, Inc.
The editors were Cathy Dilworth and Claudia A. Hepburn;
the designer was Barbara Ellwood;
and the production supervisor was Thomas J. LoPinto.
The Murray Printing Company was printer and binder.

**between patient
and
health worker**

1234567890MUMU79876543

Library of Congress Cataloging in Publication Data

Dorroh, Thelma L   date
   Between patient and health worker.

   "A Blakiston publication."
   Bibliography: p.
   1. Medical personnel and patient. 2. Sick—
Psychology. I. Title. [DNLM: 1. Allied health
personnel. 2. Interpersonal relations. 3. Patients.
W21.5 D716b 1974]
R727.3.D67   610.69'6   73-17154
ISBN 0-07-017644-2

contents

preface

This is a nontextbook, which means that technical language has been avoided and that much of the teaching is from the experiences of patients and health workers. It is written for the health worker who wishes to learn how patients feel about and react to illness and the health care system and who desires to improve his care of patients and his communication and interaction with them.

The basic objective of this book is the achievement of better health care through improved relationships between health workers and patients. Specific objectives are:

1. To teach the health worker to recognize that patients' attitudes and behavior can be understood and evaluated
2. To enable the health worker to realize how his background, experience, and self-image influence his feelings toward patients
3. To help the health worker realize that his attitudes and behavior toward patients can be changed
4. To aid the health worker in recognizing that awareness and modification of his behavior plus better understanding of patients' behavior will result in improved communication and interpersonal relationships, which in turn will lead to better health care
5. To emphasize that the personal dignity and self-respect of both health worker and patient can be preserved in an institutional setting

Technically, the term "health worker" can be applied to anyone who works in the health field, but the author especially addresses those health workers frequently referred to as nonprofessional, subprofessional, paraprofessional, or ancillary personnel. Many of these people attain a high level of professionalism even though they may not have an academic degree. It is estimated that these health workers provide 90 percent of all patient care.

Although nonprofessional health workers are usually carefully instructed in the procedure and technical aspects of their work, they get little assistance in learning what to say to patients, what not to say, or how to understand them. They are rarely taught the relationship between their attitudes and effective patient care. Even most professionals in the health field have inadequate training in human relations, and those who are trained often lack the ability to teach others.

The conviction that the training of all health workers should include material on interpersonal relations was the motivation for writing this book. Care of the sick is a great responsibility, far too great to be treated casually. Much more is involved than meeting the physical needs of patients. Good intentions toward people and a desire to be of help to them are not enough. An understanding of human behavior is essential. In the process of gaining this knowledge, the health worker will find that patience, self-discipline, and a respect for patients as persons are basic requirements. Often the health worker will be frightened and troubled by the things he sees and hears. He may be angry and resentful over the responsibilities he must carry. If he is fortunate, there will be someone in the health care system he can turn to for reassurance and encouragement. Frequently, however, he will be alone. There will not be time to seek help before he must act.

This book will not provide answers to all the problems the health worker will face in human relations; rather, it will suggest some solutions and encourage him to come up with some of his own. A bibliography is provided at the end of the book for the health worker who wishes to further his knowledge and understanding of patients and of himself in relation to health care.

acknowledgments

I am the most deeply indebted to the patients and health workers who taught me all the important things I know about health care.

I wish to acknowledge the suggestions, criticisms, and support of the following members of the University of Missouri faculty, although none of them are to be held responsible for the content of this book: William D. Bryant, professor of economics; William M. Jones, professor of English; Dr. Warren P. Sights, director of operations, Regional Medical Program; Dr. Sherwood Baker, chairman, department of community health and medical practice; James A. Irvin, associate chairman, department of community health and medical practice; Robert A. Boissoneau, assistant professor, health services management; Ronald Aldrich, instructor, health services management; Harold Kane, instructor, health services management; Dr. Clement Brooke, professor, department of pediatrics; Dr. Marjorie Dale, medical field director, Missouri Crippled Children's Services; Jacques Admire, assistant to the director, Biomedical Information Service; and Frances C. Wurtz, assistant professor of nursing.

I also wish to acknowledge the special assistance of the following people: Ida Brugnetti, education consultant, Health Manpower, HEW, Washington, D.C.; Russell Green, professor, art department, Stephens College, Columbia, Missouri; Dr. David Jones, director of medical care studies, York Hospital, York, Pennsylvania; Dr. Lester E. Wolcott, associate dean, Texas Tech University School of Medicine, Lubbock, Texas; Dr. Omar Kenyon, chairman, department of psychiatry, Evanston Hospital, Evanston, Illinois; Martha Kenyon, former chairman, Evanston Mental Hygiene Society, Evanston, Illinois; Dr. Glenn Dorroh, internist, Lexington, Kentucky; Grace Mayberg, social worker and marriage counselor, Minneapolis, Minnesota; and Louise Hadley, Mt. Dora, Florida.

I would like to give special thanks to James Hennes, consultant for planning and evaluation, Colorado Department of Education, Denver, Colorado. Dr. Hennes helped me plan, organize, and develop the concepts I have tried to teach. His reasoned, thoughtful comments and his ability to conceptualize complex material made this book a reality.

I am particularly grateful to Al Teoli, assistant professor, medical illustration division, School of Allied Medical Professions, Ohio State University, Columbus, Ohio, who provided the illustrations for this book.

Finally, words cannot properly express my thanks to Elaine Schrader, Alice Hinson, Marilyn Lafoon, and Jerri Luthy for the typing of my manuscript and Jack Barnhouse for the preparation and organization of the index.

THELMA LEE DORROH

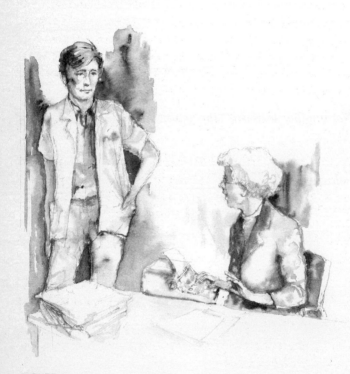

FIGURE 1

"A nontextbook," the author replies, "where most of
the teaching will be done by describing the experiences
of patients and health workers and reporting
their comments. Furthermore, you are going to help me
write it."

The health worker, young, aggressive, quick to think and to act, is standing before the author's desk.

"What kind of book?" he is asking suspiciously.

"A book designed for health workers; to help them better understand patients and how their own feelings and attitudes may interfere with effective patient care," the author, who is not so young, replies. She has strong feelings about the quality of health care and often is discouraged when she sees the unmet needs of patients. She is persistent, however. If she can arouse the interest of the health worker and teach him better ways of caring for patients, perhaps they will benefit both the patient and the health worker.

"Not another textbook!" the health worker says in a tone of disgust.

"A nontextbook," the author replies, "where most of the teaching will be done by describing the experiences of patients and health workers and reporting their comments. Furthermore, you are going to help me write it."

"Now wait just a minute," the health worker begins in alarm.

"The writing part I will do, but I need your ideas, your questions, and some of the solutions you have worked out in caring for patients."

The health worker is pleased, but he is not going to show it. "Well, I don't know."

"Will you try it? This will be a new experience for me too, you know."

The health worker was very thoughtful. "OK," he said at last, gruffly. "What have I to lose?"

1 patients and health workers

"... it's the little things. . . ."

"My sister had a terminal illness and we had little money."

"My little girl had to spend many months in a body cast."

"... taking everything away that's me."

"A different world from any that you have ever known."

"Tell me, doctor, I want to know."

"Communication, it ain't."

"No one has a right. . . ."

"I'm afraid. . . ."

"Will it hurt, Mommy?"

"I won't be deformed."

"They all have their own problems."

1 when people are sick

The health worker came into the author's room and eased himself cautiously into the chair beside her desk. He seemed a little subdued.

"About this book," he said. "How are we going to start it?"

"Why not start with how people feel about being sick?" replied the author smiling at him as she took out a pen and yellow pad from her desk drawer.

The health worker thought this over and then asked, "How are we going to know how they feel?"

"We'll ask them."

When people are sick small problems become big ones. Little worries become mountains. Decisions are hard to make. There is anger at one's helplessness, irritation with pain and discomfort. There are many fears. There is fear—close to panic—that the truth about the illness is being withheld. There is also fear, to only a slightly less degree, that one will never regain his identity as a person but will remain forever a number on a medical chart.

it's the little things

One patient said:

You will laugh. And I can, too, now. It was a small thing, a fly, as a matter of fact, which almost caused me to leave

the hospital. It kept buzzing around my face, and there wasn't anything within reach to kill it with. I rang the bell and asked the nurse if she would kill it. She looked insulted and walked out of the room. After a while, an attendant came in with some clean towels. I asked her.
"I don't see no fly," she said, and she, too, walked out.
It got to be a test of wills. I rang the bell again. No one answered. I waited a little while and rang again. No one answered. I waited a little while and rang again. No answer. By that time, I was furious. I got out of bed, although I wasn't supposed to, and with some effort bent down and picked up my slipper and killed the damn thing. And then, of course, I was caught climbing back into bed, and there were words and, well, I almost left the hospital. I might have if I hadn't felt so terrible. After that, I was treated as if I were a psycho case. . . .

Another patient agreed:

Yes, it's the little things that really get to you when you are sick. The medical care, the nursing care, as far as I was competent to judge it, was good enough—nothing great, you understand—but all right. Things like the cleaning woman who always banged my bed with her mop bothered me. I was pretty uncomfortable for a few days and any jar or movement was—well, uncomfortable. I didn't want to say anything to her. Poor soul! Probably no one had ever told her to be careful about such things. And I didn't want to make any trouble for her, so I didn't say anything to anyone. But every time she cleaned my room, "Bang" that mop would go against the bed. Well, I survived. But it was things like that. . . . And, oh yes. Do you know that they really do wake you up out of a sound sleep to give you a sleeping tablet. I thought that was one of those stories people made up. . . .

Little things! Little things! But so important when one is ill. In many ways the world of the sick is strange and sometimes out of focus. For every patient it will be different, because patients are different and because each has his own way of "coping" with disaster. The illnesses patients have will be different and reactions to them will vary. One person's fears will not be those of all patients. The thing that brings comfort to one patient may be the very thing that is most distressing to another. The wife of a patient in a nursing home said:

> *The attendant who cares for my husband comes into his room in the morning with his fists up and dances around as if he were boxing. "Well, Colonel," he'll say, "Ready for a round this morning?"*
>
> *My husband will snarl some obscenity and they are off. While the attendant shaves and bathes and dresses him, they keep up a running conversation, the attendant teasing, making provocative comments about the baseball game the night before, or the lousy race to be run this afternoon. They both argue about the points of the horses and my husband, swearing happily, will always take the opposite side of the argument. I suppose this is called "man talk." I'm just ignored.*
>
> *After my husband is dressed and in his wheelchair, the attendant lights his cigar and goes off with some parting shot like, "See you around, buddy," and my husband is smiling and looking more like his old self. One day after the attendant had left he said, "Know why I like that guy, Marie? He's the only goddamned bastard around here who treats me as if I'm not laid out on a slab with crepe on the door. Hell! Marie," he said pleadingly, "we both know I'm not going to make it. But we don't have to dwell on it all the time."*

But another patient in the same nursing home said of the same attendant:

> *I can't stand that grinning ape. He comes in and keeps up a constant chatter about things I don't know and couldn't care less about. I have learned to shut him out and make only a grunt now and then. He never listens. It takes me an hour to get relaxed and calmed down after he leaves. Oh, he's efficient enough. But we aren't all like that cigar-smoking colonel down the hall. . . .*

effect of first impressions

The first thing a person notices when he becomes ill and seeks health care—be it in a doctor's office, a hospital clinic, or a nursing home—is the appearance of the building and its furnishings. From these he seeks to find some clue as to the kind of people who will care for him. Sometimes appearances are misleading. One woman went to a faith healer's office in Los Angeles "out of curiosity," she said:

> I walked into this beautifully furnished waiting room with a carpet so thick that you sank up to your ankles in it. Nothing had been overlooked to make the patient feel welcome. The attendant was a pleasant, motherly looking woman, who greeted me warmly. I don't recall the colors of the drapes and walls, but they were subdued and pleasing. Of course, there was soft music. By the time I was called into the faith healer's office, I was so bemused, I paid little attention to the rather cursory examination and, still in a trancelike state, paid the stiff fees without question. And I call myself an intelligent woman!

Most places which care for the sick are not that attractive and sometimes the patient's or his family's reaction is so strong that they never recover from the first impression. A woman said:

> My sister had a terminal illness and we had little money. When she needed nursing home care, our doctor referred us to a home out in the suburbs. I took her there one afternoon. It was a big, old, brick building with steep marble steps, worn from many years of use. Over the entrance, carved in marble, were the words, "Home for Incurables." I looked to see if my sister noticed. She was staring up at them, but there was no expression on her face. She said nothing and neither did I. The interior was equally gloomy and grim, with high ceilings and dark painted walls. The patients were in their rooms and seemed to be quiet and silent. The personnel from the matron on down were unsmiling although, I presume,

efficient. But we didn't stay. When I told the matron that I would let her know later about taking a room there, my sister gave a quick sigh and clutched my arm.

We found another place. It wasn't very fancy. It was an old building, too. But there weren't those dreadful words above the entrance. It was noisy. Patients in wheelchairs were in the halls and there was much chatter; yet, the ill patients had their privacy. It was the personnel, I guess, more than the building which attracted us. They were pleasant, not offensively bright and cheery, and they seemed to always know how to individualize the patients. My sister was there until she died.

Death is never easy for us. But I think my sister was as comfortable as it was possible to be.

unattractiveness of health care institutions

Many health care places are grim and unattractive. In recent years a number of nursing homes and continuing care centers have been built. Most of them are well built; attention is given to the furnishings and the whole appearance is generally pleasing. The quality of care in these places is harder to evaluate, however.

In many of the big-city clinics and teaching hospitals, one gets the impression that the buildings are designed for the convenience of the staff rather than the patients.[1] The rooms are arranged so that the electrical outlets for all the equipment needed to care for patients these days are readily available to the staff. It never seems to occur to anyone that this often means that the bed is arranged so that the patient cannot look out the window. Even if the view does not particularly appeal to anyone, it breaks the monotony for the patient. There is never a clock in the patients' rooms, yet time becomes an important factor, especially in the long night hours.[2]

[1]Esther L. Brown, *Newer Dimensions of Patient Care*, part 1, Russell Sage Foundation, 1961, p. 34
[2]Ibid., p. 36.

There is seldom color in the furnishings of health care centers, except in the privately financed ones. Perhaps it is an obsession with dirt that causes most people to feel that white—which is not a color, according to artists—is more sanitary and attracts fewer germs.[3] For whatever reason, most hospitals or clinics have white, beige, or grey walls. Some have experimented with colored sheets and gowns, but most places have white walls and white or grey furniture. There are no rugs on the floor and, of course, no curtains.

A few years ago a children's ward in one of the teaching hospitals was painted brown—dark brown—so the marks of little hands wouldn't show. Another teaching hospital, however, hired a "color expert" who had the walls and corridors painted in bright, cheerful colors and had storybook characters and animals splashed on the walls and in unexpected places—such as on a crib or behind a door—in the children's ward. Some of the hospital staff didn't like the colors. Why? They found it hard to explain. "It doesn't seem like a hospital. It doesn't seem as clean looking with all this color." But the patients and their families loved it. As one mother said:

> *My little girl had to spend many months in traction. She had been a very active child and this was very hard for her. She quickly tired of her toys and picture books. Then she got interested in the paintings on the walls and together we made up stories about them. I think this helped her to pass the time more than anything. When I visited her, she would tell me about the story she had made up about "Bunny" or "Tiger" the night before when she couldn't sleep.*

Most places where the sick are treated are cheerless,

---

[3]This attitude about color applies not only to health care facilities. It is deeply rooted in our culture. After World War II, a young contractor purchased several blocks of suburban land and put up rows of cheap little houses all exactly alike except that they were painted different colors. As cheap and flimsy as they were, there was something charming and gay about them. They sold more quickly than his competitors' houses. However, three years later, almost all the houses had been repainted white.

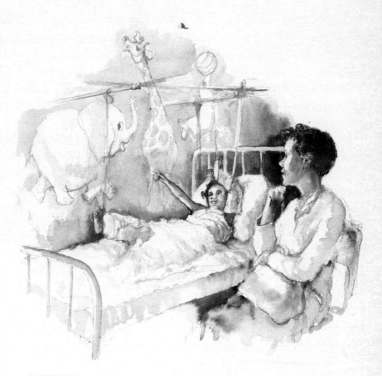

FIGURE 2

"My little girl had to spend many months in traction,"
one mother said. "She had been a very active child
and this was very hard for her.
She quickly tired of her toys and picture books.
Then she got interested in the paintings on the walls
and together we made up stories about them."

ugly, and without comfort or beauty. It almost seems as if we
don't want our sick to be too comfortable. *It is as if we wanted
to punish them for being sick.*

depersonalization

It's not only the appearance of the buildings—"that institutional look," someone called it—that upsets some patients (not all)

but also the kind of depersonalization that goes on—"taking away everything that is me." When a patient first goes to a hospital or a clinic he is given a number. If he is admitted to the hospital, all his personal belongings are taken away from him, and he is clothed, whether male or female, in the same sexless white garment. He may be allowed to have his own robe or bed jacket.

One young patient insisted upon wearing her black lace bra, even to sleep in. "I have to have something that makes me feel like a person, not like a thing." In nursing homes or continuing care centers, the rules about belongings are not usually so strict, but there are limitations. No pictures on the walls and only a few personal possessions are usually the rule. "It's too hard to keep track of them," one matron said. "We don't have enough personnel."

In one nursing home an elderly patient who was blind and who had always been a friendly, sociable person had a candy jar on the table by her bed. When visitors came to call, her first response was, "See my candy jar? Do have a piece of candy!" Often the candy jar was empty but her guests never told her. The matron was concerned:

> *I have thought of saying she couldn't keep it, because the other patients slip in and steal the candy when she is asleep. But it's terribly important to her. It's her "security blanket." And I can't be too severe with the other patients. They have so little.*

In the hospital the patient is seldom called by his name: "The doctor says you may sit up for an hour," or "It's time for your x-ray treatment." One patient said bitterly:

> *One attendant who looked after me used to come in and say archly, "Do we need to go to the bathroom, now?" or "It's time for our bath." Really, she did. And she was so hideously cheerful.*

Even the professional staff depersonalized the patient. When the physician in a teaching hospital makes ward rounds, he may say, "Now *this* patient . . ." or "*This* lady was brought in this morning with a compound fracture . . ." One patient commented:

> *You don't know whether they don't bother to find out what your name is, or whether it is just a habit they get into. Whatever it is, it gives you the strangest feeling that you no longer have any identity. Sometimes you feel like the old woman in the nursery rhyme who awoke to find her skirts had been cut off. And she cried, "Is this I, or not I?" It's really weird, you know. A different world from any you have ever known.*

problems in communication

When people are sick, old ways of communication fail. Families smile falsely—avoiding the patient's eyes—evading his questions. "Don't worry. You will feel better tomorrow," they say brightly in an unnatural voice.[4]

A patient will say, "Tell me, doctor. I want to know." Usually the physician will tell him simply and directly all he wants to know. However, communication between a doctor and his patient is a complicated matter. Sometimes the patient who says, "I want to know, doctor," really doesn't want to know, for many reasons—perhaps out of fear of not wanting to face unpleasant things. The doctor has to know his patient well enough to be able to give him the information he needs to know—in doses he can tolerate. Frequently, both the doctor and the patient feel frustrated. One physician said:

> *If I say I don't know, my patient thinks I am keeping something from her. If I say I am waiting for all the reports on the tests to come in, she's sure I am putting her off. It is often easier to make some noncommittal statement and get out of the room quickly. But that doesn't make the patient happy either.*

---

[4]The voices of most persons who enter a patient's room take on a forced cheerfulness. One training manual for nurse's aides stresses, "Always be cheerful." For some patients, this is good; others find it irritating.

Another doctor seemed to have a special gift for communicating with his patients. A nurse who had known him for many years said:

It's really difficult to describe just what he did. He'd come into a room where his patients and possibly some of the family were waiting, and he'd sit down and sigh, run his hand through his hair, sigh again, and say, "Well," and then squirm around in his chair. By this time he had the family leaning forward, breathlessly, and the patient hardly breathing, so intently was she waiting for his next words.

Finally, she'd say, "What is it doctor—is it? . . ."

"Oh, no! No!" the doctor would say, "Nothing to get into a tizzy about. It's just, well, there are two or three things you can do and I just don't know which to recommend."

I used to call it his "helpless act." He'd get the family and the patient so involved in helping him make a decision that they forgot to be frightened and he would feed little bits of information as they could tolerate it. Sometimes it was the patient who would tell him what should be done. The patients thought he was great. He had a lot of imitators among the medical students, but none was very successful.

But communication when one is sick is more often frustrating. As one patient said:

Communication, it ain't. I decided that when I was sick, the only person who gave you an answer when you were a patient in the hospital was the man in the business office. When I asked him what my bill was, he answered loud and clear. But the others! People would come into my room—some of them I didn't have any idea what they were doing there—and they'd ask all kinds of questions, some of them very personal.

One little guy with a beard came bouncing into my room one day. He was smoking a pipe—terrible smell. He sat down and started firing questions at me so fast I could hardly manage to ask, "Who are you and what do you want?" He gave me a superior smile and said, "I'm doing some research."

"Well, you can just do it somewhere else," I told him, "and take your smelly old pipe with you."

He got mad and said I'd get his data messed up. I didn't care. I wouldn't answer any of his questions. He stormed out and I didn't hear any more from him.

I know patients do ask silly questions sometimes, like "What time is it?" or "When will they bring my dinner?" But it's because we're sometimes lonely—or bored. We just want a little conversation with someone who is pleasant and who treats us as if we were persons. Patients know that the staffs in hospitals are always busy. They tell us often enough! But it doesn't take much time to smile and say a pleasant word.

lack of privacy

Then there's privacy, or rather the *lack* of privacy, to cause distress for patients. Most persons have a certain amount of seclusion in their daily lives and think little about it until they have an illness and have to stay in a hospital or some other health facility. There are other people who have little opportunity to be alone. They may live in a crowded tenement or in a house filled with people of all ages or sizes. While they may not like the crowded conditions in which they live—indeed, they may strongly resent them—when they are ill, privacy becomes acutely important.

In crowded hospital clinics or doctors' offices—and they all seem crowded these days—it is difficult to preserve the patient's privacy. And sometimes the staff forgets how important this may be to a patient. For example, an elderly man is called up to the nurse's desk and given a paper carton. He is told that a urine specimen is needed and that he can go down to the men's room in the next corridor. All this is within the sight and hearing of other patients. For some individuals, this is embarrassing.

One patient, a middle-aged woman, told of having been referred to the hospital to undergo a series of tests to rule out a possible tumor. Of course, she was frightened. Her husband was concerned and did many little things to make her feel more comfortable. One day he brought her a red silk "shortie nightgown." She was wearing it on the day an attendant came in, bundled her into a wheelchair, and without telling her where they were going, wheeled her down the hall to the x-ray department. There she waited, along with several hundred patients, for two or three hours before she was seen. She was self-conscious and embarrassed and said she kept tugging at her gown hoping it would get longer. Then she had to go to the bathroom. And there was nothing to do but to get up and parade across the waiting room to the rest room. She said she was angry at the attendant, at her husband for having bought such a frivolous garment, and in fact, at everyone. "If only the attendant had given me a robe, or even a sheet to put over my knees. The only good thing about the experience was that, in my anger, I forgot to be scared for a little while."

Privacy to patients means not only privacy as far as their person is concerned, but privacy in what they share with their doctor. It is often difficult for patients who must share a room with one or more persons to have to discuss intimate details in front of them. Patients have come to believe that whatever they tell their doctor is confidential and that no one but the doctor ever sees their medical chart. If they stop and think, they realize that other people also have access to their chart, but this they can accept if they are members of the professional staff.

A lawyer told of an experience his aunt had:

She was a very private woman, my aunt. She was ruthless in her business deals, she was rough talking, and in her behavior she had her own code and lived by it. She fooled most people, even her doctor.

"She's taking this pretty hard, having this hysterectomy," I told him.

"Nonsense. I've known her a long time. She's a powerful woman. She can take anything."

"Underneath she's just a quivering mass."

The doctor looked at me as if I were becoming unhinged and walked away without bothering to answer me.

I knew my aunt better than he did. I had seen her when her husband died and when her dog got sick and had to be killed. She was, as I said, a very private person who kept her feelings well concealed. They only spilled out when she ran into a situation she could not control.

After her surgery I saw her several times. She was quiet, listless, and too polite. I was worried. On the third or fourth day after surgery the doctor called me. He sounded exasperated.

"The nurses tell me your aunt has been found crying several times. And, he added, "she's running a fever too," as if it were my fault.

"I'll see what I can do," I said.

She wouldn't talk with me at first. Just turned her head away and ignored my questions. Finally I said,

"Now see here, Aunt Martha . . ." and to make a long story short she finally told me what was bothering her. In the first place the doctor wouldn't let her be "just female" and talk of her fears about the surgery. He saw her as a strong woman and he expected her to be strong and silent. I couldn't help much with that but I did spell it out for the doctor, and I also spoke with one of the nurses whom I knew quite well. The other problem was more complex. The day before her surgery a young man had "bounced" into her room (her words) and in an offensively cheerful voice asked if she would like a prayer said for her. She replied if she wanted anything like that she could ask for it. He responded by saying he meant no harm, but that he knew that women who were going to have a hysterectomy were *usually pretty upset. How did he know this? He'd read it in her chart, was the reply. She must have blasted him at this point because he apparently got a little angry and said "There are a lot of people besides the doctor and nurse who read the charts. It's not all that secret." This had really upset my aunt. She was extremely sensitive about having the surgery and had told no one but myself about it. The thought that everyone in the hospital knew what kind of operation she'd had really undid her. It was a small community and she was certain it would be all over the town. "I feel as if I had been stripped naked. No one has a right to read my chart except the doctor and the nurse," she said firmly.*

I will agree that my aunt was unusually sensitive about the surgery and that perhaps her feelings about the invasion of her privacy were not entirely reasonable, but this was the way she felt and I did not argue with her. Instead, I let her talk the whole thing out. And when she concluded by blowing her nose vigorously and said, "I shall sue the hospital," I knew she was going to be allright.

However, I could not help a feeling of regret that students in the health field, not just seminary students, but students of all kinds, nursing students, medical students, psychology students—you name them—have to do their learning on patients. I wonder how many times patients are hurt by thoughtless, insensitive remarks or by invasions of their privacy.

the fears of patients

Patients have many fears. Unexpressed, fear may affect the patient's response to his illness and also influence his interaction with the staff. In turn, the staff does not always identify the patient's behavior or comments as expressions of fear, and even if fear is identified, they do not always know what to do about it. The health care staff is more comfortable with obvious matters such as setting a broken leg, treating bedsores, taking x-rays, or changing a bed. However, some degree of fear is present in every patient and the health worker needs to learn how to recognize it and to learn what responsibility he has in treating fear.

unreasonable fears

And there are fears—unreasonable, unrelated to fact—which may be part of a particular illness or just there waiting to pounce upon a patient and engulf him. A social worker told of making ward rounds one day with the psychiatrist, the residents, and the head nurse.

In one of the rooms an elderly man was crouched in a corner of the room with his face to the wall. He was trembling.

"What's the matter, Mr. Reilly?" the psychiatrist asked gently, helping him to his feet and leading him to a chair.

"I'm afraid," was all he could say. "I'm afraid."

And indeed, he looked afraid. His face was ashen, he could not stop trembling, and he stared around without seeing any of us. He clung to the psychiatrist's arm.

The latter spoke softly, "We will give you something to help you, and in the meantime. . . ." He turned to the nurse and said, "Get someone in here to stay with Mr. Reilly until he is feeling better. Now!" he commanded, as the nurse hesitated.

We waited until the attendant came. The psychiatrist did not say much, but he held the patient's hand. When the attendant came, the doctor transferred the patient's hand to his and said, "Stay with Mr. Reilly until he is feeling better. Let him hold onto you if he needs to. You don't have to say much. Just speak quietly and gently."

Outside the patient's room one of the residents asked, "What was he afraid of?"

The psychiatrist shrugged. "When he is feeling better, he may be able to tell you, but probably not. Unreasoning, nameless fears are more common than we think. Sometimes it's because of the kind of illness or because of too much alcohol or drugs. The most important thing is that the patient has contact with someone who cares about him."

fear of pain

"Will it hurt, Mommy?" the child asks as they go to a doctor's office. Adults want to know this, too, although they may not always ask. Studies have shown that some people are more sensitive to pain than others, and that people who are tense and anxious may feel pain more than when they are relaxed. In the army when recruits are brought in for their vaccinations, it has often been observed that while the frail-looking fellow may walk through the line without a quiver, often the big "muscles type" collapses in a faint at the sight of a needle. Women are reported to be able to endure more pain than men, but this is questionable. Whatever the illness, there may be fear and concern about pain and the wise clinician will say, "This may hurt a little," or "If it hurts too much we will give you something. . . ." He never lies to the patient about the pain.

Patients who go to a clinic or hospital for an examination and treatment are often afraid of some permanent disability. Sometimes the fear of being disabled is not realistic. Sometimes the disability, if there is one, is only temporary. At other times there may have to be a choice between permanent disability and life itself. An example of this is a patient admitted to the gynecological service for some minor complaints:

fear of deformity

A young, rather pretty woman was assigned to a four-bed ward. During a routine examination a mass in her breast was discovered. When biopsied, it was found to be malignant. The young resident went in to tell the patient and urged her to have surgery while hospitalized.
"What does that mean?" the patient asked suspiciously.

Since he was deeply interested in his work, the resident explained in some detail and even took out his pencil and made a drawing which he gave her. So absorbed was he in his explanation that he was unaware of the patient's lack of response and when she pushed away the drawing and it fell to the floor, he picked it up and put it on her lap again. When he finished talking, the patient said,

"No."

"What do you mean?" *the resident asked.*

"I won't have it."

"Don't you understand this may save your life? It's a very simple operation."

"I won't be deformed."

"But lots of women. . . ."

"I don't care what other women do . . ." *and she turned her head away.*

The resident tried pleading with her and reasoning, but she would say no more. He was a little angry.

"I'll come back later and talk with you," *he said coldly and walked out of the room.*

When he returned that evening, the bed was empty.

"Where is she?" *he asked the other three women.*

They didn't answer him. Just looked at him. Finally, one said, "She's gone."

"Where?"

"She left the hospital."

"Why? She was . . . this, well, this could be serious."

The three women said nothing. They avoided looking at the resident. At last one shrugged her shoulders and said, "It is maybe, that you were not simpatico. . . ."

The resident stared at her. "Now, what does that mean?"

The woman shrugged her shoulders, "Ask her."

"Now, how can I?" *the resident snapped. He glared at the three women. They looked at him with stony faces. He left the room again.*

"I guess I goofed on that one," *he told his chief.*

"You did, indeed. You'd better try to find the patient."
The resident tried, but the patient had vanished. She had moved and no one could or would tell him where she had gone.

It is usually not the responsibility of the health worker to handle these kinds of fears with the patient or try to reassure her. If it is not his responsibility, he should not attempt to do so. Usually it is the responsibility of the patient's physician, even when he handles it badly. However, the health worker needs to know that patients have such fears and sometimes, because he may have the confidence and trust of the patient, he can persuade him to try to make the doctor understand how he feels.

"I'd feel silly telling the doctor about the stupid things I am afraid of," one patient said. Nevertheless, if it is a fear, it is something that she should talk over with her doctor. If the health worker cannot persuade a patient to do this, perhaps he can consult his superior. Depending upon his relationship with the physician, he might say, "Maybe you'd better spend a little more time with your patient to find out what's bothering her."

Don't be like the nurse's aide to whom a patient confided her fear of impending surgery. "Oh, my goodness," she exclaimed. "Don't let them operate on you! I had the same trouble and they operated on me. And I've never felt right since."

fear of getting well

Then there is fear of getting well. For patients who must return to a world of problems without solution, recovery from illness can be traumatic. This is the kind of patient a hospital staff finds most difficult to understand. "But he's well! Why doesn't he want to leave? Is he crazy?" No, not really. Perhaps frightened or confused. Often he is alone. Like Mrs. Salerno, for example:

"I think my back pain is coming back. And I know I have a fever," she tells the doctor.

"Nonsense! You are just fine. Sure you'll have some pain at times. After all, you aren't so young anymore, but you don't need to be in the hospital."

"But doctor, I'm not able to take care of myself yet. Maybe next week. . . ."

"No. We're going to discharge you today."

Mrs. Salerno begins to cry. "But, doctor . . ." she cries to his retreating back. She is still crying softly and hopelessly when the attendant comes in to help her dress. "You . . . everyone . . . has been so nice. Just to have someone to talk to . . . you don't know what that means. . . ."

"But, dearie, don't you have any family?"

"No, there's no one."

"But isn't there anyone in the apartment house to look after you?"

"They all have their own problems."

When she is dressed, Mrs. Salerno picks up her bag and walks unsteadily down the hall. She does not see her doctor and the nurse coming down one of the side corridors. They watch her go down the hall and out of sight. The doctor says, "I don't understand that kind of patient. What was I supposed to do with her?"

The nurse shrugged, "She'll be back."

"Yes, she'll be back. Half dead from malnutrition or from an overdose of barbiturates. . . . And I won't know any more than I do now what to do."

"You can refer her to social service."

"I suppose so, but. . . ." He sighs in exasperation and walks off.

Patients, especially those in mental hospitals, sometimes find the only security they have ever known in a hospital. They resist all efforts to discharge them. If they are discharged, they find some way of getting readmitted. One patient has been placed in a nursing home a number of times, but after a short while she always becomes so disturbed she has to be returned to the hospital. Once she is readmitted, she becomes a model patient. Asked why she doesn't like the nursing home, she has many complaints. "They don't have enough staff. The food isn't as good as the hospitals. And the doctor never comes to see me." Penal institutions have had a similar problem. Former inmates, in some cases, have deliberately committed a crime in such a clumsy manner that they were almost caught and returned to prison.

There have been attempts to try to help such people: the patient and the prisoner. Some of them, such as the Halfway House programs, have had a limited success. However, there seems to be no satisfactory solution for the person who knows better than the staff that he cannot "cope" with the outside world. If there were more people trained in how to listen perhaps more solutions could be found for this kind of person. Different methods of treatment might be useful. Certainly the punitive approach does not help.

fear of dying

Fear of dying may be so deeply rooted that it may never be put into words. Indeed, the patient may be only half aware that this is the cause of his uneasiness, but almost every patient has known or heard of someone who had his kind of illness and died of it.

"This is only minor surgery," the physician may say, but to an apprehensive patient, there is no such thing. Any surgery is of great importance to him. "I know the doctor is not telling me everything," he may confide to the health worker. This may be true; sometimes his physician has *not* told him everything, deliberately. His assessment of the patient leads him to believe it would not be wise to do so. There are, of course, patients who will be frightened no matter what anyone says to them.

Certain kinds of illness are especially fear producing. At one time, before the discovery of lifesaving drugs, tuberculosis was a very dangerous illness. It is not to be taken lightly even now. Earlier, one sometimes heard a patient say, "What's the use of going to the hospital? I'm going to die anyway and I want to be with my family." Cancer is a frightening disease. There are other illnesses equally dreadful which do not seem to carry the same degree of concern.

It is possible that some of the educational material on television, radio, and in the newspapers and magazines have created as much fear as understanding. Unless one knows the patient very well and knows how he handles fear, it may go unnoticed. Some of the ways in which it may be expressed are: by being irritable and demanding; by crying; by excessive animation and talkativeness; by being unusually quiet and preoccupied. It is important to know a patient well and have some understanding of the meaning of his behavior.

SUMMARY: Details, often insignificant, are important to a sick person. The loss of identity as a person and the lack of privacy assume a special meaning. There are many fears, expressed or unexpressed, when one is ill.

ASSIGNMENT: Reread each example in this chapter. While some illustrate interaction by the professional, you decide how you would have handled each problem. What would you have said? What would you have done? What have you learned about the feelings of people who are sick?

"Maybe this isn't my bag."

". . . I treated her just as I would my own child."

"It doesn't hurt *that* much!"

"I get hooked on the families."

"The end of the line."

". . . how alone most of them were."

"I felt as if I were on trial."

"Middle-class patients are so meek."

"Feeling is . . . the spice or seasoning of a personality."

2 not only patients react to illness

The health worker and the author were looking over the notes they had taken for the first chapter.

"Some of that stuff really shook me up," the health worker said uneasily. "Do you think health workers feel the same way?"

"I think we will find they feel just as strongly as patients, but perhaps about different things. Caring for the sick can bring out all kinds of emotions."

"Well," said the health worker without much enthusiasm, "I guess we had better get started. I knew," he added darkly, "I shouldn't have started this. It's going to be one big headache."

health workers react to the things they hear and see

Not only the patient reacts to illness. All the people who have responsibility for caring for him, health worker or professional, have feelings, spoken or unspoken, about sickness and patients. The medical student imagines he has the symptoms of every disease he studies. The psychology student wonders if he is not like the patients he is testing. As he goes about his assigned tasks in a busy clinic or hospital, the health worker will see many things which will be upsetting—accident victims brought into the emergency room, patients in great pain, patients dying, women in childbirth. If he works in a mental hospital he will hear and observe patients saying and doing strange and unpredictable things. If he works in a nursing home he will see old people disoriented—wandering around without clothing, soiling themselves as does a child, crying and laughing inappropriately. Everything he sees or hears he will react to.

Sometimes the health worker will hear other staff members making comments to or about patients which are rude, show disrespect or even hostility. He may even observe neglect or mistreatment of patients. To these things he will also have some reaction. Hopefully, he will *never* view mistreatment or neglect of a patient with indifference. But what he does about this may depend on a number of factors: his position, his immediate superior, his own personality. *Whatever he does, he must take care that the patient is not frightened or upset by his action.*

Let us look at some of the ways in which feelings may affect patient care. Here is an example of anger expressed inappropriately by a staff member and a husband and how it was handled.

health workers' feelings about patients
feelings of anger

A patient with an asthma attack was brought into the emergency room by her husband. She was having a great deal of difficulty in breathing. Her own doctor was out of town and when a strange physician appeared, he took one look at the patient and turned angrily to the husband. "Why wasn't this patient brought in before this?" The husband, a volatile fellow, beside himself with anxiety about his wife, exploded. "We've been trying to get someone to see her since early this morning." The two exchanged heated words across the patient's bed. She could only wave her arms helplessly. A nurse, passing by, took in the situation, stepped into the room, and said icily, "Your patient, Doctor!" Then she patted the husband on the shoulder, said "We will take care of your wife," led him to the door, and closed it after him. Later the patient commented, "I just wanted to tell both of them to shut up or go do their fighting somewhere else."

Yet that same physician, the patient reported, was wonderfully kind and understanding when she called him a few weeks later. She had been invited to visit her children for the holidays, but because of the difficult time she had been having she was fearful of going that far away from her physician. "I think the trip would do you good," he told her, "if you don't overdo it." "I know physicians in both the cities you plan to visit and I will give you their names and also send them a summary of your chart, listing the medications you are taking. But let's hope you don't have any further trouble."

"I like him much better than my other doctor, who's a pretty cold fish. Probably he'd had a bad day, the time he saw me in the emergency room."

There will be times when the health worker will find himself filled with anger toward a patient or a member of the patient's family. The anger may be justified. But showing his anger by word or action is *not* justified. This may take rigid self-discipline on his part, but this is something he must learn. He may be angry with his associates or his superiors. How he manages his feelings will vary with the situation which provoked his reaction. Again, much will depend upon the kind of person he is, but his anger toward superiors or associates must not be expressed before the patient.

feelings of dislike

There will be times when the health worker will find he dislikes caring for certain kinds of patients. This is not surprising. Health workers have such varied backgrounds and experiences that they are not always equipped to handle all the situations they have to face. One social worker whose entire case load was nursing-home patients told her supervisor:

I don't know what to say to them. What can I say? They're all going to die, aren't they? You say it's wrong to put on the bright and cheerful act when people are old and sick. Well, I don't feel like doing that but what can I do? They are always complaining about something—their food, the attendants, that their doctor hasn't been to see them. I think some of them make up complaints just to get some attention. They are always wanting to touch me. I can hardly bear that. One old woman said, "You're scared of us." When I said I wasn't she just kept nodding her head and repeating, "You're scared of us. Yes. Yes." Maybe she's right. I think the whole thing scares me. Maybe, well, maybe this isn't my bag.

Yet other health workers have found experiences in the nursing home which were satisfying to them. One woman, a practical nurse said:

I guess I like it because it's kind of a low-pressure place, if that means anything to you. It's not the rush-rush you find in a hospital where everyone is so busy and it's so crowded. You get to know the patients here. You know what one likes to eat and another one doesn't. Some patients like a back rub at night, and others just want you to tuck them in bed and leave them alone. Some of them are cranky and bad tempered but it's hard on them, having to live in a place like this. They miss their families and miss being able to go about and do as they please. Of course, I can go home to my family after my work is done. Maybe that's why I don't mind it so much.

The health worker is not expected to like all the things he is required to do. And if he is honest with himself he will know he is more comfortable with some kinds of patients than with others, but he knows he must learn how to care for all kinds of people. And as he gains in understanding of sick people and acquires more intimate knowledge of himself, his tasks will become easier. It will no longer be a question of like and dislike but rather of how he can do what needs to be done in the best way to help his patients.

too much feeling

Liking a patient too much may be just as much of a problem for a health worker as disliking him. Sometimes before he quite realizes what is happening he is overinvolved. This sometimes happens on a children's ward where the emotional appeal of a sick child is so great that the health worker responds as if it were her own, resenting the interference of anyone else who attempts to care for the child, and especially resenting the parents who are made to feel like intruders. Often the health worker is unaware of how deeply she is involved. Even when her supervisor points it out to her, she may protest.

"But I treated her just as I would my own child."

"But she is not your child. She has a mother."

"Ha! You should see her mother. She's so stupid she doesn't know how to care for her own child."

"Perhaps you can teach her some things."

"Teach her! You should see her!"

It is not easy to learn the degree of involvement with a patient that is the right amount but not too much. Young doctors sometimes pay more than the necessary amount of attention to a young and pretty patient. A young social worker went through a stage of caring so much about each of her patients that it was almost as if she were defending them against the rest of the world. All their problems became hers and she battled fiercely with anyone who appeared to reject them. At the end of a day she was exhausted. So was her supervisor. Eventually she learned that sometimes she was doing more harm than good, that certainly she should care about her patients but that she must learn "to help them help themselves."

too little feeling

It is better that a health worker be overinvolved with his patients than underinvolved. There are some health workers who appear not to care about any of their patients. They do what has to be done without show of interest or concern. There are some people who seem to be incapable of, or who have little capacity for, warmth or positive communication with others. They are the "loners" and one wonders why they chose a job where emotions are such a large part of any health care activity. There are others who are afraid to show their feeling, fearing it is inappropriate. Young people in many professions—teaching, nursing, medicine, social work—go through a stage of "being professional" which they assume means showing no emotion or warmth. But as they learn more and gain in some personal security, they dare, timidly at first, to show friendliness, concern, or normally appropriate emotions. They learn to their surprise that often their interrelationships improve remarkably.

feelings of superiority or of power

Sometimes underinvolvement assumes a different face. The health worker seems to imply by his manner a feeling of superiority to the sick and helpless people he cares for. He may say to a patient, "*I've* never had a sick day in my life," or "I don't see why you are making such a fuss over a little thing like that! It doesn't hurt *that* much!" The people who care for sick people are in a position of control, often of decision making, and sometimes there is misuse of this power.

feeling overly sympathetic

The health worker who has experienced severe illness himself may be more sympathetic and understanding of the sick person's needs, but not necessarily. It will depend upon how he himself adjusted to illness. If it was a very frightening experience he may be overconcerned, overattentive. An overanxious mother is a good example of this kind of response. If the experience with illness was more pleasurable than painful, and sometimes this may be the case, for instance, in a person with a great need to be taken care of, a nurse's aide for example, may be impatient or resentful of her patients. "They never had it so good. All they have to do is lie there and let other people wait on them." The nurse's aide may say this aloud or she may think it and show how she feels by the way she handles her patients. She may slap a pillow down, jerk a wheelchair too abruptly, ignore a patient's buzzer, or spend so much time talking about her illnesses, her operations that the patient can hardly get in a word.

health worker's feeling about certain kinds of illnesses

Certain kinds of illnesses create apprehension in many health workers. "I could never work with mentally retarded people," one may say. "It's too depressing." Or another will say, "I don't know why, but people who are deformed or crippled just, well, they just upset me." Fortunately, there are many people who do not respond negatively to the handicapped, the mentally retarded, or other sick people. Others may start out with uneasiness or distaste, but with experience become deeply interested in the very people they at first rejected.

the brain-damaged

A physical therapist in a home for retarded children said:

When you first come here, you just want to turn around and run as fast as you can. But after you are here a while it gets to you. At first all the children seem pretty hopeless and then you begin to see that one child can do some things, very simple things, and another child can do something else. You get hung up on trying to see what they can learn. It's surprising sometimes, if you just take the time and have enough patience. And I am always interested in what caused these children to be handicapped. I try to take

a very careful history, hoping that some of them will hold
some clues for the research staff. There's such a lot no one
knows about the causes. And then there are the families of
these children. I get hooked on them. Parents have a lot of
emotional investment in a child and when something
happens and the child is handicapped, it's a terrible
experience for the parents. All their dreams destroyed!
They need a lot of help before they can come to some kind
of terms with the knowledge their child can never be what
they had hoped and planned for him.

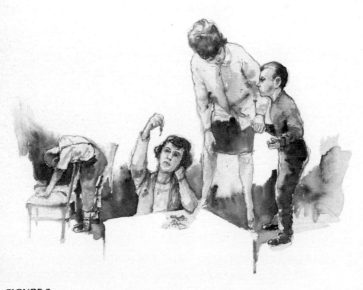

FIGURE 3

"At first all the children seem pretty hopeless and
then you begin to see that one child can do some things,
very simple things, and another
child can do something else. You get hung up on
trying to see what they can learn. It's surprising sometimes,
if you just take the time and have enough patience."

the mentally ill

A great deal of money has been spent over the last decade in educating people about the signs and symptoms of mental illness. Equal amounts of money and time have been spent trying to deemphasize the stigma which still seems to cling to the patients and their families. Some of the attitudes are deeply rooted in our culture. Folklore and mythology play their part. The drug therapies of the past decade have helped return many patients to the community. Other types of therapy have helped many of the patients return to a useful and productive life. But as in all other types of illness, much still needs to be learned, much still needs to be taught. Once, reflecting the communities' attitude of "sweeping them under the carpet," mental hospitals were built in isolated areas. Now the trend is to locate them near teaching hospitals or the larger communities. This means it is easier to utilize community resources, also hire and keep personnel. But still there are shortages, particularly in health workers. Caring for the mentally ill lacks the drama, and immediacy, found in other hospitals or outpatient clinics. *And probably not enough emphasis has been placed upon the importance of the health worker's contribution to the treatment of the mentally ill.* In some areas mental hospitals have developed very good programs, described as the therapeutic community, in which all members of the staff participate. Successful as these have been, not only in aiding the patient but in improving the morale of the staff, they have been costly experiments and have not generally been accepted.

the chronically ill or acutely ill

The chronically ill, as do the mentally ill, lack the appeal which attends the care and treatment of the acutely ill patient. The latter receives the best of medical care and should, and probably it would be impossible to maintain for long the high intensity of effort and attention which accompanies his treatment. Physically and emotionally it would be too exhausting.

Unfortunately the routines required for caring for the chronically ill are often repetitive and boring. In busy hospital clinics an asthmatic may be greeted by the health worker with the comment, "Oh you're here again." Another patient will be asked, "Now what do you want?" Both professional and health worker find these patients uninteresting. The patient senses this. Sometimes he will say apologetically, "I wish I had some exciting disease for you to work on."

In nursing homes, where most of the patients are classified as chronically ill, are found examples of some of the poorest kinds of health care. There are exceptions, where excellent care is provided, but in many of the homes, the health workers have no training, there is little supervision, and worst of all, they sense and quickly learn to imitate the attitude of the rest of the staff. They make many mistakes in caring for the patients, not because they are mean spirited, but out of ignorance. Perhaps the most demoralizing thing of all is that the health worker learns that no one cares what he does as long as the ordinary routines are maintained. It's the attitude of the staff that marks the difference between poor and good health care and some of the best care is sometimes found in poorly equipped homes. One example was a nursing home in the Middle West. It was located in a semirural community in what had once been the county poor farm. Apparently through faulty construction, because the building wasn't really too old, it was considered dangerous. Over a period of two or three years, several citizens' groups and the state health department tried to get it closed. The county court was slow to take action on condemning the place because they had no other place to put the patients. And to everyone's surprise, the families of the patients, the patients themselves, and the staff all strongly resisted any change. While all the reports had noted that the patients seemed well cared for and happy, the significance of this was not recognized. Letters to the editor poured in, the families criticized the health department and the citizens' groups for snooping, and the county judges, with an eye on an upcoming election took no action. The nurse director spoke ruefully about the situation.

It's true the patients here do get a kind of care not often found in some of the larger nursing homes. I think it's partially because the patients and staff have the same rural background. The staff knows the kind of life these patients had before they came here; they often know the patient's family. There is a kind of family feeling here between the patients and staff. They plan little parties together; there is a lot of joking and kidding, and the patients do improve remarkably here. The families like to visit. But knowing the shape the building is in, I don't sleep well at nights. On the other hand if we had a brand-new shiny building, I wonder if we'd have the same kind of give and take between patients and staff. A building shouldn't make all the difference . . . but I wonder.

the dying patient

There has been an unusual amount of writing on this subject in the past few years in professional journals for nurses, physicians, psychiatrists, psychologists, sociologists, social workers, and ministers. Although this material is written for the professional, some of it is useful for the health worker. Certainly, both professional and health workers find caring for the dying patient one of the most difficult of their tasks, and the one they handle the most poorly. There will be further discussion of this in one of the subsequent chapters, but the health worker needs to understand that while the *management of their own feelings is one of the most difficult things they will ever have to learn*, it is especially traumatic when caring for dying patients and their families. A young and untrained social worker tells of her experience on a cancer ward of a big city hospital.

I had reason to feel my supervisor did this out of hostility, since she knew my mother was dying of cancer. Relations between us had not been happy for some time. I was angry and dismayed. I was not sure I could go on that ward and control my own emotions. But I determined I would give no sign of how I felt to the supervisor. And I made myself go up to the ward. The first sight of it almost undid me, accustomed as I was to many tragic scenes. It was a big, gloomy room with beds lined up along both sides. Around a few beds were screens, which meant a patient was dying. Most of the cases were terminal. As I walked around the ward I was sure most of the patients knew this. I was stiff and awkward at first, so rigidly was I trying to manage my feelings, but the need of these patients for some human contact was so great that I soon was deeply involved. Their requests were simple: a glass of water, a phone call to a relative, or a letter to be written. Some few patients seemed to have already withdrawn from this world and made little response to me, but most patients seemed to want someone near them. Sometimes without any exchange of words they would reach out and hold onto my hand.

Consciousness of my mother's illness remained a dull ache deep down in my heart, but I managed somehow to function in spite of it. It wasn't because I was all that noble, but because I had to. The experience took its toll. It was never easy to go on that ward, but it became less difficult. I learned from the patients some things which I think helped my mother. One thing I will never forget is how alone most of them were. Their visitors, if they had any, did not stay long, and the hospital staff, professional or nonprofessional, hurried in and hurried out again. Often I was the only staff person on the ward.

health workers' feelings about certain social classes

Certain social classes of patients will evoke reactions from the health worker. In one hospital the financial classification for each patient is indicated on the face sheet. Anyone who handles the chart can see this. "Oh, he's a welfare patient," a health worker may say scornfully, or "He just gets Medicare." In this same hospital, unwed mothers or indigent patients are housed in a dormitory for two or three weeks, depending upon the nature of their illness and the kind of care they need. But they are not allowed in the dining room until everyone else has eaten. For breakfast, they must wait until nine o'clock, and for lunch until one o'clock. They line up outside the dining room to wait for the time they will be admitted. All the hospital staff must pass them on their way to and from the dining room. To the unobserving, these patients seem to be unconcerned. They laugh and talk among themselves. They appear unaware of the curious, sometimes hostile, and sometimes sympathetic looks of the staff members as they walk past them. However one unwed mother said:

> I felt as if I were on trial—everyone knowing who we were and staring at us. The experience canceled out a lot of the good things that happened in that hospital. For the most part, people were kind and didn't make you feel you were different, or that they blamed you for what happened. But standing in that line, waiting to get something to eat, well, sometimes I couldn't eat once I got into the dining room. And sometimes I would say I wasn't hungry and go and get a candy bar.

One cannot but wonder at the corrosive effect on the staff who witnessed this scene one, two, and sometimes three times a day.

Some health workers dislike caring for black patients; others, for any kind of "foreigner," but not all react negatively. A clerical worker found her job in a community health clinic an exciting experience.

> I like working here. I think I would find any other job a dreadful bore after this one. As the young say, "This is where the action is." It's true. The patients speak their mind. If they don't like the kind of health care they get, they say so. Middle-class patients are so meek. They take all kinds of insults, and never say a word. But not so,

these blacks, or these Mexicanos. They let you know. And their vocabulary, it's wonderful. I should write down all the new words I am learning.

The staff here is different too. Most of them are here because they want to be, and they really get involved. In the drug program, the staff elected to be on call twenty-four hours a day. I would just like to hear the screams in the hospital where I used to work if anyone ever suggested that they be on twenty-four-hour call.

health workers' acts of neglect or cruelty

Congressional committees, citizens' committees, and other investigative groups have documented material describing instances of cruelty and mistreatment of patients, particularly in nursing homes or mental hospitals where often there is too little supervision, overcrowding, and inadequate or poorly trained staff. There are reports of patients being oversedated, beaten, starved, and given emetics or cathartics as punishment. Many of the nursing homes where such reports come from are not licensed by the state but operate only because there are not enough beds in licensed homes to meet the demand. But even in the better ones examples of mistreatment can be identified. In one prestigious nursing home, very expensive, an attendant left a hot-water bottle in the bed of a paraplegic too long. The patient had little or no sensation in her extremities and before the error was discovered she had received second- and third-degree burns. In that same home a visitor overheard an attendant cursing an elderly patient who had apparently soiled herself. Asked if he reported this incident, he said, "Oh, no. I didn't want to get involved."

Incidents such as these should never be allowed to happen. If they do, the health workers responsible should be dealt with promptly. Unfortunately, such acts are not always reported to the proper authorities, perhaps because the witnesses are afraid or, worse still, do not care. Think of the malignant effect upon the health workers, an effect which may influence their own treatment of patients, if such behavior to patients goes unchallenged.

the origin of feelings and attitudes

Many references have been made in this and the previous chapter to the *feelings* of the patient or the health worker. Not as much reference has been made to *attitudes,* but they too have their place in health care. Attitudes, the way people think, are the intellectual extension of the way people feel. Both terms are often used interchangeably, but in this book the greatest emphasis will be upon feeling. If one's feelings are appropriate to a situation, his attitude will generally be appropriate also. Not always, but most of the time.

Feeling is the quality which gives spice and seasoning to a personality. Without the capacity for feeling there would be no ability to feel pleasure or pain, joy or sadness. An incident which occurred some years ago illustrates this.

A conference was held at one of the state hospitals. Psychiatrists, neurologists, psychologists, social workers, and residents in psychiatry attended it. The guest speaker had perfected a method of treatment for acutely disturbed or intractable patients called a frontal lobotomy. *A more popular term was "ice pick operation." The surgery was relatively simple and did not involve much danger for the patient. The fibers of the frontal lobes which controlled the emotions were incised. The speaker was most enthusiastic, emphasizing the small amount of danger and the fact that patients who were inclined to destructive or violent behavior were rendered tractable and no longer presented a problem of management to the institutions. (Then, as now, institutions were short of staff and were even more crowded than now, this being before the discovery of the various drug therapies.)*

As climax to his speech, the speaker had a group of

patients, some twenty-five in number, ranging in age from sixteen to seventy, brought out on the stage. They stood there, quietly, passively, and as the speaker singled out certain ones and gave details about their previous behavior, they made no response. Their faces were without expression. They did what they were told to do, but without emotion or initiative.

Later the group visited the ward and were shown other patients who had had this surgery. All of them were obedient, tractable, quiet; but there was no animation, no response to the visitors, positive or negative. "My God," one of the psychiatrists said, "They're Zombies!" Someone else said, "This reminds me of one of those horror movies where a mad scientist destroys the souls of his victims." No one at that meeting ever forgot that experience. It is good to know that this type of operation is seldom used today.

personal and environmental experiences

Yes, one should indeed be glad he has the capacity to feel, even though feelings, poorly handled, can create problems, especially in the health field. But if the health worker has some awareness of his own feelings and some understandings as to why he has them, he is well on his way toward managing them so that they will not impede good health care. The goal is *knowledge of feelings plus understanding of them.* This is not easy to achieve, because why we think and feel as we do is often (1.) rooted in experiences formed early in life; (2.) influenced by the attitudes and behavior of those close to us; or (3.) affected by the environment in which we live. What we are and what we become is often a combination of these three elements. For example, if the mother of a sick child is herself frightened and anxious about illness, the child senses this from the way she holds him, the way she hovers over him, her tone of voice as she talks to the doctor. He then becomes fearful and anxious and this interferes with the way he responds to illness.

Another mother who can manage her feelings so that she speaks calmly, yet tenderly, and makes herself move quietly and do whatever has to be done with little fuss and apparent unconcern will help her child to be better able to cope with the strange and frightening experience of being uncomfortable and even in pain. The first mother is unaware of the effect of her own fears on her child. The second mother is very much aware of this and while she does not deny to herself that she is afraid she manages her feelings so her child is not influenced by them. A child seeing the love and attention his mother lavishes upon his baby sister when she is ill comes to feel that illness is a pleasurable experience, wherein he will get all his mother's affection. Still another child, raised by his grandmother and her sister, had a different experience. A neighbor of them says:

> *They were great pill takers, those two. A different colored pill for every ache or pain. And the grand time they had comparing symptoms, and what the doctor said, and what so-and-so did when she was sick. No wonder the poor child grew up thinking that there was a pill for any and all of his problems "if only he could find it."*

cultural experiences

Cultural influences on illness and health deserve a separate study, but the health worker should be aware of the effect upon himself and his patients of such forces. There is still secret admiration for the stoical approach to illness. The little boy who sits quietly in the dentist's chair and utters not a whimper is called "Daddy's brave little boy" and gets praise from both his parents and the dentist. But let him give a healthy cry if the dentist hurts him and he is called a "crybaby" and quickly senses the disapproval of his parents and sometimes the dentist. There have been studies of women in childbirth which indicate that the woman who screams and yells during delivery may actually come through the experience with less trauma to herself and her child. But even though the staff in the delivery room knows this, the "sweet, suffering woman" still gets more than her share of approval.

Some of our attitudes about illness seem to be changing, however. In the Victorian era and for some time thereafter, it was considered gentile for a woman to be fragile and delicate. "To be ailing," "to feel puny," or "to have the vapors" were some of the expressions frequently heard. When a neighbor reported, "Martha is feeling poorly today. She had one of her spells again," all the women would nod their heads gravely and with a certain satisfaction. Martha had achieved a kind of social status with her illness and they respected her for it.

But men, if they are sick, receive less sympathy and attention. Illness in men is often associated with weakness and unmanliness. The little boy who is too frail to play rough and strenuous games frequently is teased and even treated with cruelty by his playmates. A little girl who is delicate fares much better. Not too long ago some women learned quite early in life that they could control the members of their families quite successfully with their illnesses. The mother who took to bed with a headache or had a "heart attack" if either her children or husband flaunted her authority is an example of this. Some men also used this method, but they were never as successful as the women.

The son or daughter who gave up marriage to devote his entire life to the care of an ailing parent once received praise from the minister and indeed the entire community. "What a wonderful son, or daughter. How fortunate his parent is to have such a child." If the child of such a parent rebelled, he met with disapproval. Now the parent who attempts to use illness to control her family receives little sympathy. "It's a shame what she's doing to her family. Someone ought to get her to a psychiatrist." And probably they should. Her children are more likely to receive pity than praise.

Perhaps we are moving slowly and uncertainly toward some healthier attitudes toward illness and health care. But in isolated communities old patterns remain, and in other areas, attitudes may not be better than they ever were, but merely have a different focus. The message for the health worker is that he must be aware of the influence his environment has had upon him and he must also be aware of the significant forces in the patient's environment.

SUMMARY: In this chapter are narratives which describe health care from the viewpoint of the health worker. Emphasis has been placed upon the importance of the health worker's feelings and attitudes as they affect patient care. Some of the elements which may cause these reactions and some of the factors which may influence the way the health workers feel and act were also discussed.

ASSIGNMENT: Think of experiences you have had in which you showed intolerance, anger, or insensitivity toward patients. You need not share this knowledge with anyone, but look at it carefully and decide how you might have handled the situations. Ask yourself why you acted as you did. Was it because of the environment in which you grew up? This assignment is difficult but try to complete it.

2 the patient the family and the illness

"I'm not a psychologist, Ma'am!"

"Largely a matter of semantics. . . ."

"I wonder if the doctor knows what he is doing."

". . . as if we were gods."

"What could we have done?"

". . . no one will ever know how scared."

"It's a part of getting well."

"I felt apart from everyone."

"And so finally."

3 how patients deal with illness or injury

The health worker was indignant. "What's this got to do with me? 'How patients deal with illness or injury.' I'm not a psychologist, Ma'am."

"Heaven, forbid! Your job is caring for patients, but how can you do this unless you know something about people and have some idea of how they adjust to illness or injury?" The author sighed, "I think I have said some of this before."

"You have. But go on. I'll at least listen."

With this questionable assurance, the author proceeded:

A patient responds to illness or injury in the same manner in which he has learned to respond to previous stressful situations. To describe this in another way, each patient has his own life style and has developed his own ways of coping with unpleasant or painful situations. The degree or intensity of his responses may vary, but they follow a pattern. It is not always possible to know how a patient has previously dealt with stress, but he provides some clues by the way he relates to the staff, by the questions he asks, and as significantly, by those he does not ask. His mood, the things he does, all give some hints as to the way he has learned to react to trauma.

While each patient has his own reaction pattern to illness or injury, there seem to be certain elements or a certain series of reactions common to most traumatic situations. Elisabeth Kübler-Ross has identified these for the dying patient. In her eloquent and compassionate book, *On Death and Dying,*[1] she has listed five stages the patient goes through after he learns that he is dying. She describes these as:

denial and isolation
anger
bargaining
depression
acceptance

Lester Wolcott, Chairman of the Department of Rehabilitation and Physical Medicine, University of Missouri Medical Center, uses somewhat the same technique in discussing the reactions the rehabilitation patient experiences in adjusting to his injuries. His list is somewhat different from that of Dr. Kübler-Ross but he is identifying, as does she, the emotional reactions of patients to illness or injury. He groups the stages in the following manner:

anxiety
anger
hostility
depression
normal

No attempt will be made to discuss these two arrangements in detail, always a risky business and particularly so in Dr. Wolcott's case, since his material is not yet published, but the author felt that the focus of these two physicians on the emotional aspects of illness was closely related to the emphasis of this book, i.e., the importance of knowing how patients feel. Stimulated by the material presented by Drs. Kübler-Ross and Wolcott, the author has developed still another order for the emotional steps patients pass through in adjusting to illness or injury. Some of the same concepts as those pre-

---

[1]Elisabeth Kübler-Ross, *On Death and Dying,* Macmillan Company, New York, 1969. (Although written for the professional in the health field, this book should be required reading for all health workers.)

sented by Drs. Kübler-Ross and Wolcott are included but this list is adapted to meet the particular needs of health workers. Furthermore, the health worker should be able to identify the different stages in most of the patients he will see. The author's description of the emotional stages through which the patient moves before he reaches some resolution or acceptance of his illness is presented as follows:

fear or anxiety
affront
anger
depression
resolution

Largely a matter of semantics, the health worker should feel free to experiment with this arrangement of the emotional stages a patient experiences, describing them in his own terms. The important thing to be stressed is that patients have emotional responses to illness and that these responses will vary with individual patients and will change. Now to consider these stages as the author perceives them:

"I'm afraid"   fear or anxiety

Any stressful situation generates some fear or anxiety. Depending upon the kind of stress, and depending upon the manner in which the individual has learned to cope with stressful situations, the reaction may be mild or intense. The student who takes an examination may be only slightly uneasy, or very anxious. Minor illnesses or injuries may create more concern than they seem to warrant. "Is this more serious than the doctor is telling me?" "What if I get an infection?" "Is this going to be painful?" The patient may not voice his concern. But he watches everything the doctor does and listens carefully to any comments which are made.

Remember the patient in Chapter 1 who was able to say only "I'm afraid," and could give no name to his fear. Another patient, told she should have a thyroidectomy, repeatedly asks, "But doctor, do you think this is really necessary?" She stops the nurse, the resident, and the social worker and of all them she asks the same question. At home she talks of nothing else. "I wonder if the doctor knows what he is doing?" "Do you think I should have this operation?" She asks anyone who comes in. But she derives little comfort from any of the responses she gets. Why is she so fearful? No one asks her why or what she is afraid of.

During the polio epidemic of 1951, a fourteen-year-old boy was admitted to a ward already crowded with polio victims of all ages and sexes, men, women, and children. He did not seem acutely ill but he appeared dreadfully frightened. When it was necessary to put him in an iron lung, his fear seemed to increase. All the staff, the doctor, the medical students, the nurses, a psychiatrist, tried to reach him in some way and reassure him. But it was as if he were deaf. He heard no one. He died within a few days and it seemed he had died of fright rather than of the illness. History about him was meager. But it was learned he was an adopted child, abandoned by his parents. His foster mother never visited him in the hospital. The staff was left with the question: "What could we have done? Surely there should have been some way of reaching him."

"why me?"   affront

Stress implies and may actually be a threat to one's self-esteem, one's person. It may cause embarrassment, feelings of anguish, of pain, physical or mental, or even death. Stress of any kind evokes the reaction, "Why should this happen to me? Why me?" The student confronted with a difficult examination may think, "Other profs don't give such tough exams. Why should mine have to?" The motorist arrested for speeding thinks, "Why did that cop pick on me? Others were doing the same thing. Why me?" A patient responds in the same way. "Why did *I* have to get sick? I've never had a day of sickness in my life. Why should I have a stroke now?" Often not expressed, this feeling of insult is usually present in illness or injury. It is as if we thought of ourselves as gods, not subject to the indignities or injuries of mortals.

"I was mad at everything—and everybody!"
anger

Anger is another reaction to stress. If the stress is relatively mild, as in the case of the student confronted with a stiff examination, perhaps not mild from his point of view, but still not an earthshaking event, the reaction may be milder than anger, irritation perhaps. This may be true of the motorist also—he may be violently angry, but more than likely he will view his arrest and probable fine as a "damned nuisance, but not a matter of life and death."

For patients, again depending upon the nature of the stress and their own life style, the response may be severe or so insignificant as to be unnoticed. It is, however, a necessary step in the patient's adjustment to his illness. One woman described her experience in the following manner.

I feel an utter fool when I think back on that time in the hospital when I was so mad, mad at everything and everybody. It was after the accident when I first realized I was in a body cast. I was scared—no one will ever know how scared. I was certain I would never walk again. I was convinced my doctor and my husband were lying when they said I would be all right, in time. At first those words "in time" didn't come through to me. Not until I realized I might not get up and walk out of that place in a few days, did I really begin to sweat.

"How long?" I asked my husband one day.

"What did the doctor tell you?" he said, not looking at me.

"I'm asking you."

"Well, these things take time. After you get out of the cast, you'll have to have all kinds of exercises. But you are going to be all right."

"How long will I be in this cast?" I said, suddenly so angry I almost choked.

"Six months," he said, and after one frightened look at my face he fled.

It's hard to describe how I felt then and it doesn't make sense. I couldn't move in that cast, but I wanted to kick something. I wanted to throw something and would have if there had been anything within reach. I wanted to scream, but the only thing I could do was cry.

It was at about that time the nurse came in. Jim had probably sent her. I was still crying and she was of no help. She was cheerful. "You're going to be all right. Don't worry."

I didn't need cheerful people just then nor did I need to hear any platitudes. I was rude to her. In fact, I was simply obnoxious to everyone in the next few days. Nothing pleased me. Even my doctor.

"You are one of the fortunate ones, you know," he said one day. "You might have been an invalid for the rest of your life."

"Six months is a lifetime," I snapped.

He didn't say anything, just looked at me thoughtfully and I felt dreadfully ashamed but wouldn't say so.

Not then, but later, he said, "It's all right to be angry. You have had a bad time."

I began to cry, "I have been pretty awful." But he interrupted me, "We are used to it. It's a part of getting well."

Not all the staff recognize that anger is as the physician said, "a part of getting well." It will always be difficult to understand and accept the fact that seldom is there anything personal in the patient's anger. The paraplegic who smears feces on the wall is not doing it to "get back at the nurse" but because he has no other outlet for his misery and frustration. The patient who curses the attendant, complains about the food, his doctor's neglect, or the "nurse who wakes me up to give me a sleeping pill" will always be difficult to tolerate, but as one nurse said, "He hasn't given up and I'd rather deal with an angry patient any day than the one who turns his head to the wall and responds to no one."

"at the bottom of a deep well"   depression

Depression is a fourth reaction to stress. Psychiatrists will tell you that depression often occurs if there is no satisfactory outlet for anger and for many patients, especially those with chronic illnesses, there is no release. The patient's environment may be such that anger is met with strong disapproval, or the patient's own personality may inhibit his expression of anger. For many reasons, depression is present in most illnesses or injuries. It is a term often misused and misunderstood, but one the health worker must recognize if he is to properly identify some of his patient's symptoms. Usually tears are one expression of depression, and they may be, but we also find tears expressing anger, in both children and adults, or a combination of anger and depression as illustrated by the woman in the body cast.

Tears may indicate joy or pain, or in highly excitable people, tears are a response given to many situations. "She seems to have a built-in spigot which turns her tears on and off on any and all occasions," one medical student said disgustedly of the above kind of patient. On the other hand, the tears of a stroke patient may be a physiological reaction rather than depression. As a result of the stroke, many of his responses may be inappropriate; his sudden laughter, explosive anger, or unexpected tears do not always indicate strong emotional reactions.

There is always danger of self-destruction, suicide, in any depression. The health worker's responsibility may be only to report any unusual comments or acts of the patient, but this is a great responsibility, because he may be the first one to note some significant change. A patient sometimes conceals his feelings from his physician or the rest of the staff. "I'm feeling just fine," he may say, smiling broadly when rounds are made, but the minute he is alone, bursts into tears.

Some patients will talk about being depressed. Often they use slang or colloquialisms. They may say, "I'm feeling down in the dumps." "I was so depressed, I cried all night." "Nothing seems to matter to me." "I don't care whether I live or die." Sometimes the patients will use the past tense as if the depression was no longer present. "I felt apart from everyone." "I felt too miserable to cry." "I felt as if I were at the

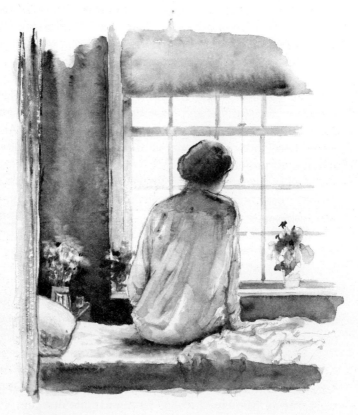

FIGURE 4
"I felt as if I were at the bottom of a deep well."

bottom of a deep well." One needs to know the patient in order to determine the significance of such remarks, and they should be evaluated in relation to whatever else the patient may be saying or doing.

In certain illnesses depression seems always to be present. This is especially true of chronic illnesses. One health worker commented that it seemed as if patients with crippling arthritis always had "a dark cloud hanging over them." The diabetic patient is often depressed and at these times sometimes will stuff himself with forbidden foods, a self-destructive act which may have serious consequences. Both Dr. Kübler-Ross and Dr. Wolcott seem to feel that depression is most likely to occur when the patient first faces the reality of his situation. In many patients, however, "the dark cloud" seems to be present most of the time.

An abrupt change in mood may signal depression. For example, the patient who has been sullen and hostile may suddenly become unnaturally cheerful and animated. Another patient, the one who is usually friendly and outgoing, becomes silent, listless, eats poorly, refuses to participate in any activities, and in general seems preoccupied or "turned in upon himself." It is well for the health worker to keep in mind that *any sudden or marked change in mood should be reported to the nurse or physician-in-charge.*

"and so finally"   **resolution**

A Pennsylvania-Dutch woman had a disconcerting way of ending her conversation with the phrase, "And so finally." In most instances there comes an end to stress. The crisis does not remain a crisis. Some resolution is achieved and the person adjusts to it. Our student gets his examination paper back and he passed or failed. The stress is over and he moves on to the next crisis in his life. The motorist pays his fine, and he too moves forward, ready to forget an unpleasant experience. For one patient the end of stress may be recovery from his illness.

For another it may be seeing at last the face of his fear. The paraplegic now knows what his future will be and grim as this is, there is a sense of relief. From somewhere, somehow, the individual dredges up resources to cope with the disaster which neither he, nor no one else, knew he had. Very unbrave men can show remarkable courage when once they come face to face with reality. However, if a resolution of the stress cannot be achieved or if the patient is unable to accept the reality of his situation he may remain in an anxious, depressed state. If this should last too long, he may need specialized help, perhaps from a psychiatrist. . . .

> *The author stopped, put down her pen, and pushed the manuscript away. Turning to the health worker, she said, "My task, you know, is not easy. I don't want to frighten you with too much knowledge, but I want to give you enough to lead you into wanting more. I don't want you to lose confidence in what you are doing, but neither do I want you to be satisfied with the way you are doing your job." She sighed, "I can't tell whether I am succeeding or not. . . ."*
>
> *The health worker did not look at her. He looked at the floor. He was subdued. "I don't know what I think. I just don't know." "But," he added with a flash of his old belligerence, "I am not quitting just yet."*
>
> *"Shall we proceed?" asked the author.*
>
> *The health worker nodded. "Tell me what I am going to do with all this. . . ."*
>
> *"I shall try but first let us look at the human variable."*

the human variable

Remember, all patients don't march through each of these stages in the same, one-two-three order. This fact is at once the joy and the frustration of working with people. No two are exactly alike. Each one has had a different life experience. Two children born to the same parents do not have exactly the same environment. The first and oldest child will be treated some-what differently than the younger child, and he in turn will respond differently than his older sibling. Some studies have been made of identical twins which suggest that they respond to similar experiences in the same way, but these studies have been challenged, because who can say two environments are the same.

The anthropologist Mark Zborowski postulates that there is a cultural difference in the way people respond to pain, that "patients of Italian and Jewish origin tend to be more emo-tional while experiencing and expressing pain"[2] than the Anglo-Saxon, whom he defines as the Old American "whose ancestors have dwelt in the United States more than three generations."[3]

Illness may only accent a lifetime of anger, anxiety, or depression. Learning about people and why they do the things that they do is an endless process, and no health worker can be expected to become an "instant expert," but whatever he learns will be of value and not only help his patients but enrich his own life and make his job one that is more than a series of dull, dreary tasks.

what does the health worker do?

In going over the material in this chapter, the health worker will note that he already has acquired some ideas as to how patients may be helped, but some further detail may be useful. The health worker should try to ascertain which stage of reaction the patient is in. This may not be easy but observing and listening will help. It is important to keep in mind that patients will move from one stage of reaction to another *at their own pace.* This process cannot be rushed. And indeed, sometimes real harm can be done if efforts are made to do this.

[2]Mark Zborowski, *People in Pain,* Jossey-Bass Inc., San Francisco, 1969, 239.
[3]Ibid. p. 6.

For example, to force a patient to face the fact that he may never walk again before he can absorb it may cause him to go into a state of shock. When he is able psychologically, he will look at this fact, unpleasant though it be. It's almost a question of digestion, emotional digestion. The health worker's major responsibility is to support the patient through these various stages. By support is meant the health worker's interest and concern and actual presence when the patient needs someone near him.

Sometimes the best thing a health worker can do is to say nothing but in a quiet, unobtrusive way show his concern by attending to the patient's wants, doing small things to make him more comfortable. Dr. Wolcott gives an example of a newly admitted patient who rings the call bell frequently. If the bell is ignored, or if it is answered and the health workers show impatience or annoyance, the already anxious patient may become more fearful. Actually his frequent requests, usually inconsequential ones, are his way of testing this new and strange environment. Is it hostile? Are people kind, or unfriendly? However, if the bell is answered promptly and if the health worker takes a little extra time with the new patient, his anxiety subsides and his demands decrease.

Sometimes the patient may say, "I'm scared to death." This should be accepted matter-of-factly. Responses such as, "Most patients are," or "It is frightening to have to come to a place like this" are often enough to reassure and support the patient, but if he expresses concern about particular details of his illness, the worker may say, "I'll see if I can't get someone to explain this to you."

It is futile and, if one reflects upon it, positively stupid to say to a patient, "Don't worry. You are going to be all right." In the first place how does the health worker know this, and in the second place, fear or anxiety, indeed no emotion, can be turned off at a command. This is a mistake often made, and it is frequently irritating to a patient. He senses the lack of real concern in such overworked phrases. It's far better to say nothing or to make some general comment. "There are a lot of things to get used to in this place." "Probably everything seems very strange." "Is there anything you'd like to know about this place or about what you can expect to have done to you?" The worker will have to proceed cautiously with this last question. He may be free to explain general procedures of the hospital or nursing home, but details about medical or surgical procedures will usually be explained by the physician. However, if the patient voices concern about such details, the health worker should report this to his superior.

The health worker has to conceal his own reactions. Of course he will have some. He has to be "unflappable," often under trying situations. Sometimes the patient may say or do something which strikes the health worker as laughable. But let him be very sure the patient is in a mood to be laughed at. "We are not amused," Queen Victoria once said haughtily, and a patient often loses his sense of humor when he is ill and perhaps in pain. Another patient may "laugh that he may not weep" but to join him in his laughter is not always appropriate.

Anger is, as already noted, most difficult for the health worker to accept without responding. If he can say calmly "I expect I'd be mad too, if I were in your shoes," or "It's all right to get mad. No one is going to get upset," this kind of response is far better than the overly sympathetic approach: "You poor thing. I don't see how you stand it."

Patients who are depressed make the people around them anxious and there is a rush to do something—often the wrong thing. This activity sometimes relieves the staff more than the patient. The following example describes the way one situation was handled:

> In the outpatient psychiatric clinic one day, a young medical student rushed out of his office and up to the front desk where the chief nurse was sitting.
> "What do I do?" he asked anxiously, "My patient is crying."
> The nurse reached into her desk, took out a box of tissues, and handed it to him. "Take this and go back into that room. Don't leave her alone."
> "What should I say?"

"Nothing. Let her cry. She probably needs to. When she is calmer, then you can try gently to get her to talk about why she feels so bad."

"Maybe I should change the subject," the medical student said hopefully.

"So you will feel better." And as he backed away she added sternly *"and don't try to cheer her up."*

Often this is the thing many people will try to do—"cheer up the patient" by telling an amusing story. If a patient is truly depressed this may make him feel worse. Of far more importance than the spoken word is the manner in which the health worker cares for the patient and his alertness to the small things which will make him more comfortable.

It is reported that when Dr. Spock was practicing pediatrics he would frequently write on the chart of a young mother with her first child, "Give this patient a large dose of T.L.C." If the prognosis is not good, when patients come to resolution of their stressful situation, they may need judicious doses of T.L.C. If they don't want to talk, they should not be forced to. If they don't want visitors, they should be protected from them but not necessarily left alone. More frequent visits to their room might be indicated, but never in a brash, aggressive kind of way. Low-keyed conversation, quiet and unhurried movements may be best, not the tiptoeing around or hush-hush mannerisms that one sometimes sees around the bedside of very ill patients. At such times as these the health worker needs to be unusually perceptive and must try to anticipate the patient's needs. Here, his previous knowledge and understanding of the patient and the rapport he has already established with him will be invaluable.

SUMMARY: To understand how patients cope with their illnesses or injuries is something which has to be learned anew with each patient the health worker sees. To know how to help and not create more stress for the patient. To learn not to speak, if he does not know what to say. To learn not to act until he is sure he knows what to do. To know when to get help, and quickly, for a patient. All these are skills to be learned by the health worker at the same time he is developing his understanding of patients. Not an easy task, but one which can be learned. Subsequent chapters will provide more material on how to understand patients and on ways the health worker can contribute to patient care.

ASSIGNMENT: Select a patient for study. See if you can determine by what he says or does just which stage of emotional reaction he is in. Try to decide what you have done or said which may have helped the patient and which things may have upset him.

"It's like walking a tightrope. . . ."

"Doesn't anyone ever read my chart?"

"What am I going to say?"

"What if he is unconscious?"

". . . the unexpectedness of people. . . ."

"Why can't you listen?"

"I am lonely, God-awful lonely."

4 knowledge and understanding of the patient

The health worker looked tired. "That last chapter," he sighed, "almost did me in. How am I going to learn all these things? The patient's feelings! My feelings! How am I going to decide what to do or what not to do? If I get too involved with my patients, that is bad; if I'm not involved enough, that isn't good either. It's like walking a tightrope and always falling off."

"Of course," replied the author crisply. "One falls off frequently, but then gets up and tries again."

"Well, I don't know about that," the health worker began slowly.

The author took pity on him. "That was a difficult chapter. Unfortunately there is no instant formula for teaching human interaction. This chapter, though, I think you will find much easier. We will start out with very simple ways you can learn about patients."

"That I want to see," the health worker said doubtfully.

the health worker's dilemma

As indicated in the previous chapters, the health worker is frequently confronted with the problem of communication or interrelationships when caring for patients and often has no way of knowing how best to handle them or how much responsibility to take in trying to do so. Much of the interaction with patients involves some form of communication and this is not so frightening a concept if one recalls that a person from the time of his first cry at birth is communicating. Perhaps it is more a matter of developing awareness of what actually goes on between two people rather than anything strange or complicated. If the health worker brings to health care a liking and enjoyment of people he will find the process of sharpening his skill in interrelationships a source of much satisfaction. If the health worker, however, is not easy and comfortable with people, he may find the processes of interaction painful.

Complicated as is the matter of interrelationships, certain basic steps can be taken by the health worker which will provide him with considerable knowledge and understanding of his patients. Some may be more suitable than others to the particular circumstances and environment in which he practices. He will need to choose the most appropriate. He can learn something of the patient by:

reviewing collected data
questioning
observing
listening
extending his knowledge
evaluating

collection of data

In effecting a good interrelationship and in attempting to establish good communication, whatever the circumstances, any knowledge or information which can be obtained aids in establishing the complicated and sometimes delicate means of communication with another individual.

In a social situation when two people meet for the first time, both attempt to identify some common bond of interest by asking such questions as "Are you related to Robert Henshaw?" or "Do you teach at the university?" or "Have you lived here long?" The questions may be more subtly phrased, but the intent is the same: to find out as quickly as possible something about the person just met.

A clever salesman quickly collects sufficient information about a potential prospect to aid him in selecting the approach most likely to achieve a sale. Fortune-tellers are exceedingly clever in picking up bits of information from a word, a grimace, a sharp catch of breath, which may be fed back to a client. It may seem as if a fortune-teller has read this knowledge in her client's palm. And in a way, she has.

In dealing with patients some of the more conventional approaches to communication are not only impossible, but would not be suitable. This is a different kind of relationship in which a human need is present for one party and the other is there to provide some aid or relief for that need. "Help me," the patient says in effect when he seeks medical care. "Relieve me of my sickness or make it more bearable." The health worker as a representative of health service is there to offer some aspect of that care to the patient. He must, therefore, bear the major responsibility for selecting and maintaining the most appropriate means of communication. It is an unequal relationship in that one receives and the other gives.

At the time a patient is assigned, the doctor's orders provide some necessary information. "This elderly patient needs to be fed. He is partially paralyzed." Or, "We need some blood tests before we can determine what antibiotics to give this child. We suspect she has meningitis." Or, "This patient is to be placed on a diabetic diet."

The health worker has questions he needs to have answered before he goes in to see these patients. For the elderly man, it may be, "Is he conscious? Can he speak? How severe is his paralysis? Does feeding mean tube-feeding or hand feeding?" And for the child the questions may be, "How old is she? Does she have family with her? Who will reassure her if she's afraid of me?" For the diabetic, another set of questions may shape themselves as the worker reads the order: "Is this a male or female patient? An adolescent or an elderly patient? Is this a new diagnosis? Is this patient likely to be cooperative? Has he been prepared for a dietary schedule?" The questions for all these patients are many.

Where does the health worker find the answers? One of the quickest sources is the medical chart. Usually the health worker picks up the chart and turns to the page where the tentative diagnosis and other medical information is recorded, reads it, and puts the chart away, completely unaware of the wealth of valuable data he has overlooked. Not only the health worker does this but most of the staff, professional and nonprofessional, follow this pattern. Seldom do any of them read the face-sheet data, unless they are seeking a specific piece of information; for example: the name of a possible blood donor. Yet the face sheet contains in capsule form a history of the patient before he entered the hospital. Such items as the following are listed: his residence, his sex, his age, his marital status, his religious preference, his employment, and his financial classification.

Most of the staff do not read this page. What do they do? If they need any of the above information, they ask the patient or his relatives the same questions that have already been answered. "I don't know how many times I've answered that question," a patient may remark with an appropriate amount of irritation. Another patient may ask, "Doesn't anyone ever read my medical chart?" At any time this happens, the first and most important rule for successful communication has been violated. *Never ask a patient for information which is already available.* This is a poor beginning for successful interrelations.

Sometimes, of course, it is necessary to verify the accuracy of the face-sheet data, but this can be done in such a way as to not affront the patient. For example, "I see from our record that your daughter's address is 1429 13th Avenue Northeast; did we record that properly?" This lets the patient know you have read his chart and that you want it to be accurate.

Not only does the face sheet provide useful data, but scattered throughout the chart are other useful items. The nurses' notes, also a part of the chart which is seldom read, often have excellent observations of the patient. The patient's history may provide additional information about the patient as an individual. Not all charts have a social history; but if they do, further details may be learned about the patient's environment. Significant attitudes of the relatives and the patient are often recorded in this section.

In any review of the chart a selective process goes on in the mind of the reader. He seeks the information he feels will be useful to him and scans the rest of the chart. Often with experience, the worker finds himself utilizing more of the material. After he has seen the patient, he may go back to the chart discovering that some of the material he originally overlooked now falls into proper perspective.

If a salesman had access to the information contained in the medical chart, he would be overjoyed and would know how to turn it to his advantage. This information provides many opportunities for positive interrelations. If a worker can say, "I see you are from my hometown. Probably we know some of the same people," or, "I see you are a teacher; what kind of teacher? I mean do you teach in grade school or high school?"

This kind of beginning tells the patient that the health worker identifies him as an individual. This is reassuring and gratifying. So many procedures and the very environment in which a patient finds himself when he seeks medical care tend to strip him of the known and familiar trappings[1] which have set him apart from everyone else, that have said in effect:

> *I am John Smith. I was born in St. Paul, Minnesota. I am 65, married, and have four children. I have worked as a laborer and bartender. My house is paid for.*

Most people cherish the symbols of their identity. Signposts of success or failure, they are the known and, therefore, are safer than the unknown.

---

[1] In Chap. 1, remember the patient who said, ". . . everything that is me."

asking questions

At this point the health worker may interrupt, "All right, I've read the chart. But it doesn't answer all my questions. I don't know what some of the medical terms mean and the dictionary didn't help much. I have some knowledge about this patient, but I don't know, well, I don't know what to do with it, now that I have it. . . . What am I going to say when I walk into the patient's room?"

Good questions, all of them, and there are doubtless others which are of equal concern to the health worker. What can he do? He can direct his questions to someone who can answer them. But he has to know who this may be. Further-more, he must know how and when to seek information. The person to query may be his immediate superior. Sometimes more than one person may have to be questioned. If inter-pretation of medical data is needed and the health facility has medical students, they may be the best source for this kind of information. Medical students delight in sharing their newly acquired knowledge with less informed individuals. A staff social worker may be helpful in planning the best way to approach the patient for the first time.

Obtaining needed information can become complicated if the nurse or physician-in-charge is the one to be consulted. Nurses and doctors are often busy or hard to locate. When they are approached, sometimes they are impatient and not eager to answer questions.

The worker will have to have very clearly in mind exactly what he needs to know and make his questions as brief and concise as possible. If he is sincere in his desire to learn, usually he will receive a favorable response: "I want to be sure I understand your orders." Or, "I have only one question . . ." or "I have read the chart, but is there anything else I should know before I see your patient?"

Choosing the proper time and place for his questions is equally as important as how they are asked. Never discuss one

patient in the presence of another. Never interrupt a conference, even an informal one, unless there is an emergency.

On the other hand, if the worker's question is essential to
his understanding of a patient, he should persist in spite of
obstacles until he has an answer. One health worker commented:

> *It becomes easier to get information after you know where
> to go and when to ask. As you become known, there is less
> need for verbal communication; the staff knows what
> questions you will have and sometimes they anticipate
> them by putting more details on the data sheet. Your
> questions are briefer and so are the responses as you know
> the staff and they know you.*

Now the health worker has prepared for the initial patient
contact by reading the medical chart and consulting with staff
members who are able to provide him with additional material.
He is in the process of sorting out the information he has
obtained, discarding that which seems unessential, and weigh-
ing the significance of other, sometimes contradictory, factors.
A picture of the patient begins to take shape in his mind. He
plans the method of communication he feels will be most
successful. He is eager to try it. Before he does, however, one
further step of preparation should be discussed. This is observation, or nonverbal communication

observing

Upon first sight of a patient, before even a word is exchanged
between you, what does he tell you about himself, what of the
color of his skin, his manner of breathing, his position, his
response to your presence? All these signs and many others
communicate something of the kind of person the patient is
and something about how he feels.

"What if he is unconscious?" the health worker may ask.
That communicates something of his state of health, does it
not?

Observation is used by the wise physician. When a patient seats himself beside his desk, using this kind of evaluation, a doctor makes a quick decision as to which clues to pursue in getting the patient's history. Sir William Osler frequently told his medical students to observe, record, tabulate, and communicate.

One nurse said she learned to make her own rounds when she first went on duty and that before speaking to her patients, she made a quick assessment, noting any external indications of the patient's state of health, such as restlessness, a flushed or too-pale countenance, listlessness. As she observed these symptoms, she mentally noted whether there was any change from her last observations and in following up on these she gave top priority to the gravest symptoms. She said just this quick review helped her choose the areas where she should spend the largest amount of her time.

The chief social worker in a psychiatric clinic, who had the responsibility for screening the patients newly referred, said that as she walked down the corridor to her desk she observed the patients waiting to be seen. If the patient was alert, gazing about with interest, or chatting with his neighbor, she made a mental note to put him aside until some of the other patients were attended to. She gave first priority to the agitated or tearful patients or the one who sat looking down at the floor seemingly unaware of his surroundings.

We never knew what kind of patient might be referred. Some of them were quite ill and needed attention quickly. Others were admitted to the hospital from that clinic. It would have been cruel and perhaps dangerous for them or for others to have kept them waiting too long. This initial observation was not always confirmed by my interview, but as I gained in experience, I found it useful and a reasonably accurate device.

With practice, the health worker can make observation a conscious tool to use in learning about people and how to interrelate to them.

first encounter

That first encounter with a patient is an unforgettable experience for most people in the health field. The medical student often endows his first contact with a live patient with almost mystical qualities and years later as a busy physician can relive it word for word. A social worker's first interview with a client illustrates this.

> *I will never forget my first client. I remember her name, her dress, which was blue, the warmth of her smile. I recall I was so frightened that I walked around the block three times before I dared to climb the steps of her house and ring the doorbell. My client opened the door, smiled at me gently, and said, "You must be my new social worker." She led me into her tiny living room, gave me a seat in her best chair, brought out a cup of tea and some cookies, and then sat down and led me gently through the interview I had come prepared to obtain."*
>
> *"You will want to know," she began, "what my expenses were this last week. . . ."*
>
> *I will never forget her. She taught me so much. Through her I learned more than I ever found in a book about human courage, honesty, and wisdom. When I was transferred to another agency, she wept, and so did I."*

Yes, that first encounter can be a momentous experience. If the health worker is young and inexperienced, even though he has tried to prepare himself, he will be anxious. When he meets his patient, he may well forget all he thought he had learned and blunder into mistakes out of embarrassment and uncertainty.

Another factor is the "human variable." Even though the patient may have been reported as friendly and cooperative, something unknown to the staff may have occurred which causes him to be unfriendly and even downright hostile. This something may have had no relation to the health care system or the health worker; it may, for instance, have been a fight with his wife, but his manner shatters all the plans the health worker has made to form a relationship with him.

It is well for the health worker to be prepared for the surprise potential in any patient contact. This is a challenge to his ability to make a quick reassessment and readaptation of his planned approach. "In this business you sure have to be flexible," one health worker said half in chagrin and half in amusement. "And alert," another added. "But that's what I like about this work: the unexpectedness of people," a third health worker commented. "I know that sounds stupid but if everyone always acted like you thought they would, well, I think it would be dull business." This health worker can be assured that the "human variable" will prevent the care of sick people from ever becoming monotonous.

listening

Now to turn to the art of listening. And it is an art. Many books have been written about it, at least one is included in the bibliography,[2] and many articles have attempted to define the elements in good listening.

Reflecting on his own experience, the health worker will be able to recall few people in his life who really listened to what he was trying to communicate. Most people are preoccupied with their own problems and often interrupt saying, "You think you have troubles. Well, let me tell you about mine." Others are in too much of a hurry to listen or are uncomfortable when not doing something or talking themselves. And there are some people with good intentions who have never given any thought to how essential it is to listen; how much there is to be learned in this way; how important it is to the person who is trying to talk. This is probably the single most important element in communicating with another individual.

[2]Theodor Reik, *Listening with the Third Ear,* Grove Press, New York, 1948.

One patient said of her physician:

You think he isn't listening to you. He sits and looks out the window and plays with his pencil; but when you stop talking, he writes out a prescription and hands it to you. If you ask him a question, he will answer it, but I can't tell whether he understands what I am saying or even cares. I am sure he is a good doctor, but his manner, well, it turns you off. I think of things I would like to say or ask about, but I don't. . . .

Another patient said of her doctor:

She's great. She really is. When you walk into her office, she greets you quietly, but pleasantly. And when you sit down, she asks a question or two and then puts her pen down on the desk and leans back in her chair relaxed and listens to you. Really listens. She makes you feel as if everything you say is so important she does not want to miss a word. You feel better even before she examines you. . . .

When this physician was told of her patient's comments, she shook her head and said:

My patients couldn't always say such things about me. Learning to listen has been one of the hardest things I've ever had to do. I'm naturally an impatient person. It wasn't easy to make myself sit quietly and appear relaxed. However, I've found listening is my most important diagnostic tool. I really don't have to ask many questions. Sometimes a question distracts a patient from something important that he is trying to say.

How did I learn this? Well, not from medical school, but from my patients, the hard way, through the mistakes I made. One patient yelled at me once, "Why can't you listen? I am trying to tell you something."

I hadn't been listening to him, but I didn't think he would know that. And another time a woman said irritably, "I wish you'd stop fiddling with that pencil when I'm talking with you. Are you nervous?"

She was half-right. It took me a long time to feel at ease with people. It's partially because I am a woman, I guess. Women doctors still have a hard time of it. Being a woman, however, my patients did not seem as afraid to speak their minds, and I think I learned more quickly than my male colleagues how to get along with them.

But back to listening. . . . When I was an intern, I saw a woman whom I've never forgotten. It had been one of those days when everything seemed to happen and I was dashing from one place to another, scared I'd overlooked something, or would do the wrong thing. At five o'clock I went back to my office, intending to slip out of my coat and dash out of the hospital as quickly as possible, but there was this woman waiting to see me.

I didn't like her. None of us did. We thought she was a "crock." She was always coming to the emergency room with some vague complaint or another, never much wrong with her. Always whining and complaining. I thought about slipping out the back door, but, well, I saw her. I wasn't very gracious about it, but I sat down in the examining room and because I was really terribly tired, I slumped back in the chair and didn't say much.

She started talking as she always did and I just sat there. Usually, I interrupted her. I don't know when the conversation seemed to change . . . when I began to see a different person. She wasn't a "crock" but a dreadfully frightened and distraught woman who must have been seeking, desperately, someone who could help her with some very serious problems.

I forgot my fatigue, sat up, and really began to listen. Between us, we got some real communication going. I didn't understand just at the time what had happened. Later when I thought it over, I realized that I had never really let her talk before. I had interrupted her, or showed my impatience by moving about, tapping my pencil, or flipping my stethoscope. She must have sensed my dislike.

She had great courage, that woman, to keep coming back when she had been rebuffed so many times.

This physician's ability to listen with complete absorption must have given great comfort to this lonely, frightened woman, but she went beyond this; as she listened, she evaluated what she was hearing. She heard not just the words the patient was using but what she was trying to communicate and it was to this she herself communicated when she responded to the patient.

Consider the elderly man in the nursing home who is always complaining about how bad the food is, how the attendants neglect him. These things may be true, but is this what he is really trying to communicate or is he saying in the only way he knows how to communicate, "I am lonely, God-awful lonely. Please, won't someone give me a little attention, just a crumb of friendliness and concern?"

The elderly woman in Chapter 1 who did not want to leave the hospital, "I think my back pain is returning, doctor," was not really concerned about her pain, but the doctor took her words literally and did not sense the inner urgency she could not express in any other way.

This kind of listening is not easy. It often takes a great deal of experience and study; yet at the same time some very simple, uncomplicated people seem instinctively to function on this level. An example of this kind of person was described by one patient.

I was going home the next day but I found it impossible to sleep. I was restless. I could not find a comfortable position to lie in. My head ached and my broken leg began to hurt and it had never done this before. I rang for the nurse and after what seemed to be a long time, she answered me over the intercom. I said I couldn't sleep and wondered if the doctor had left an order for a sedative. She said she would be in in a little bit.

Well, I waited and waited for her. I felt worse, I was angry and almost ready to cry. I felt completely deserted. I saw

no point in ringing again. I knew no one would come.
After a while, the attendant came in. Her round, black
face was full of warmth and concern. The nurse had an
emergency and would be here as soon as she could get
away, she explained. She smoothed out the sheets, got
some ice water, fluffed the pillow, and patted me on the
shoulder.
"I'll bet you are just worked up about going home tomor-
row."
I felt terribly ashamed of myself. "I think you are right," I
said. And do you know that by the time the nurse came in I
was almost asleep!

Children have the ability of going right to the heart of the
matter. Sometimes it is disconcerting. Fortunate is the health
worker who has this quality. For most people it will be
acquired skill.

"All right! All right!" the health worker will say. "So it's
great to listen but I still don't see where I come in." You will be
involved with the same patients the doctor sees. Your responsibilities will be different but it is just as important that you
have successful interaction with the patient as does the physician. There are studies which indicate that the health worker
may have as much as 90 percent of patient contact. There may
be times when you have many more opportunities to interact
with patients than does the professional.

when not to listen

Just as important as the ability to listen is to learn *when not to
listen.* The dietician, for example, should not encourage,
indeed should not allow, the patient to speak of very intimate
matters which are to be discussed only with the physican.
Sometimes the patient's need to talk is so great that to stop her
takes great skill and tact: "I'm sorry," the dietician may gently
say, "I am afraid I can't help you with that. Would you like for
me to have the doctor stop by and see you?" Or, "I am afraid I

can't be of much help to you with that problem, now if you have any questions about your food. . . ."

Sometimes the patient may say, "I want to tell you something, but you must promise not to tell the doctor." This seems flattering, but it can be a trap which must always be avoided. The physician is in charge of the case and whatever his relationship is to the patient, the health worker cannot take his place. He has to reply, "I am sorry that you can't discuss this with the doctor for he is the only one who can help you." Or, "Well, maybe you had better not tell me because, you know, I am responsible to the doctor. It might be something that I might have to tell him."

Sometimes the patient may express strong negative feelings about his doctor. Even though the health worker may not like him either, his responsibility is to help, not complicate his patient's life. He has to learn to be noncommittal. Sometimes he can say, "You are pretty angry with everybody right now, aren't you?" Or, "We all get upset with people sometimes" may be even better to say because it is tolerant and nonjudgmental.

extension of knowledge

Every experiment, every research project, every new probe into the multifaceted field of medical science produces facts and new information of potential use to the medical and health professions.[3]

The monkey is squarely on the health worker's back. He has to keep up with current information in the health field if he is to do a proper job. "I'm too tired," or "I don't have time to read," or "No one else does any reading," are comments most frequently heard. When the health worker has to spend long hours at tasks which may be monotonous, exhausting, and fraught with many tensions, it is easy to rationalize. There is

[3]Vernon E. Wilson, M.D., "Missouri Regional Medical Program: An Overview," Missouri Medicine, vol. 65, no. 9, September 1968, p. 719.

really little choice, however, if he is to keep up with the daily input of new knowledge and techniques. He has to read.

Sometimes boring tasks assume relevance if the health worker can see his assignment in relation to the total plan of patient care. The dietician in her training, for example, acquires some basic knowledge of the diseases in which an appropriate diet is an important factor. However, not until she starts to work does she have much opportunity to consider that other factors—rest, medication, surgery, psychotherapy—may be of equal importance in treating the patient. The technician may fail to see how his activities relate to others of equal importance; but when he can, his work becomes more interesting and he is often stimulated to seek further knowledge.

Additional knowledge may be obtained in several ways. One might be class attendance at a college or university. The health worker may find subjects of interest in the departments of psychology, social work, education, or sociology. If he desires to take courses for credit, he should, of course, seek an adviser and plan a program of study which will enable him to obtain a degree.

For many, additional schooling may not be possible, but these persons should not feel cut off from gaining further knowledge. There are the libraries, public libraries, or the county medical societies in some areas, and if one is near a university or medical school, professional books and journals are available. Today many good books come in paperback and the health worker can begin to accumulate volumes for his own private library. Most libraries have copying machines and for a small fee they will provide copies of chapters from books or magazine articles upon request.

Although this book is primarily concerned with understanding and improving interpersonal relationships, knowledge of other areas of health care can enrich and enlarge his experience. For the worker who finds many questions but few answers, more knowledge may be helpful. This must be his decision, however.

evaluation

Evaluation is the last step in the process of communication and interaction. This means the evaluation of whatever one reads, hears, observes. It means learning how to take acquired information, look at it objectively, and decide whether all or part of it is relevant to a particular situation. It means listening to the meaning behind the words,[4] and it means evaluating how best to meet the problem, what to say, and equally important, what not to say.

Evaluation involves awareness of one's own attitudes and reactions. Experience makes this method more useful. Some process of evaluation goes on in any communication with another person, but again, to make it a professional tool, one should give some conscious thought to the process.

SUMMARY: The steps outlined in this chapter provide some basic material on interrelationships. Elementary as they may seem, their successful application means much hard work. In future chapters, other aspects of communication will be considered but whatever means the health worker adopts, a question of judgment must be considered.[5] For the health worker to plod through each of these steps for every patient he will see, even if this were possible, would be inappropriate and a waste of his time.

One or more of these steps may be utilized for most patients but the health worker must decide in every situation which ones are to be considered. The severely injured patient brought into the emergency room bleeding and unconscious and the critically ill patient are examples of situations where

[4]Reik, *Listening with the Third Ear.*
[5]An example of nonjudgment is the nurse's aide whose duty it was to keep the pitchers in all the rooms filled with ice water. She did this conscientiously. All her rooms were covered. She went into a room where the physician was examining his patient. She entered another room where the patient was receiving the last rites from his priest, picked up the empty pitcher, and returned it filled with ice water.

the first priority is the preservation of life and the techniques of interrelationships may not be appropriate. Although they may not be necessary with the patient, perhaps they may be necessary for the bewildered and frightened relatives who seem to get in everyone's way at such times. At the same time he is performing whatever tasks are assigned to him in caring for a badly injured or severely ill patient, the health worker can use his ability to listen, observe, and evaluate not only in relation to the patient but to the other members of the health team. He can learn much about communication as it is used in times of crisis.

ASSIGNMENT: Walk slowly through a crowded outpatient clinic and choose one patient to study. Sitting down beside him, visit with him for a few minutes. No probing. Just concern and interest. How long has he been waiting? Is there anything that would make him more comfortable—a glass of water, a cup of coffee?

Later, when it can be done unobtrusively, talk with the nurse in charge of the clinic and learn what she knows of the patient. Then assemble what you have observed and learned about him. Do you have some idea of the kind of a person he is? What kind of education he has, what kind of work he does, how he feels about his illness? In short, what have you learned? What else do you need to know? How can you add to your knowledge of this patient?

". . . these are *my* responsibility?"

"Have you heard about your patient . . .?"

"That's the way they are, poor souls."

"Maybe you had better talk to the doctor. . . ."

"Most of these amnesia victims are phonies, anyway. . . ."

". . . do all their crying inside."

"The patient has a right . . ."

"He don't look so good, does he?"

"She was deeply religious . . ."

"What can I do?"

5 protection of the patient

The health worker was looking over the author's shoulder. He frowned at what he saw. "Are you saying there's a lot more to protecting a patient than things like keeping him from falling out of bed?"

The author was emphatic, "I do, indeed."

"And all these are my responsibility?"

"Yours and everyone else's who care for patients. But especially you. . . ."

"I know," interrupted the health worker with resignation. "Especially me, because I see more of them than most of the staff. . . ."

"You are learning," the author conceded, smiling slightly. "Now let's see just what is meant by 'protection of the patient.'"

areas where protection is needed

In the last chapter the health worker began to learn some of the means he might use to understand patients. Before we proceed with this discussion, it is important that he stop and give serious thought to how information obtained about patients will be used. "Information will be used to learn to better understand patients," the health worker will say impatiently. This is true. This is one of the objectives of this book. But how is the patient protected in this learning process? What responsibility does the health worker have in making certain that information he has about the patient does not fall into the wrong hands? How does he conduct himself when unwarranted questions about the patient are asked of him?

In health care, the *physical* needs of patients generally are met, but as learned from some of the comments of patients in the first chapter, some of the human, the personal, the feeling part of patient care is not always provided. And protection of the patient is not always identified as a part of health care. Physical protection, yes. When patients are irrational and unaware of what they are doing, they are protected from harming themselves or others.

Illness, whatever it is, leaves the patient vulnerable and not always able to defend himself from idly curious, morbid, or malicious individuals. There is not always protection from careless or thoughtless words or acts. The medical chart, that most intimate record of a patient's life, may sometimes be found in the hands of unauthorized individuals.

Protection from these acts has been assumed but not always defined. Only medical students are required to take the Hippocratic oath and then only when they graduate, not when they first begin seeing patients.[1] Requiring this oath only of physicians was appropriate as long as they had sole responsibility for patients. Now, however, many individuals with all levels of training are involved in some aspect of patient care. Perhaps some such pledge should be required of all health personnel.

carelessness or indiscretion

Granted that many of the errors made are not out of malicious intent but through carelessness or ignorance, the harm or hurt to a patient and his family may be just as great. An example of this are the two medical students who met in the hospital corridor.

[1]The nursing and social work professions also have an oath for graduates.

"Have you heard about your patient . . . Seltzer?" one called out.

"No!"

"He died about an hour ago."

"What happened?"

"Guess it was another stroke. . . . We. . . ." And they went on discussing the patient, hardly aware of the woman who walked past them while they were talking. She was the wife of that patient and was then on her way to the mortuary.

Another time, a group of medical students were having coffee in the cafeteria and were excitedly discussing an intricate operation for heart surgery they had just witnessed. Abruptly, a man at the next table stood up and said bitterly, "I suppose you know that you are discussing my daughter."

Not only medical students are guilty of this kind of indiscretion. Sometimes two staff members may enter a crowded elevator continuing a conversation. Without realizing it, they may make some comment which identifies the person they are discussing. A social worker stops a physician outside his office and so intent is she on reporting some information, she fails to lower her voice and nearby persons overhear something which may be very personal and private. A nurse fails to close the door of the waiting room when she talks with a patient on the phone. The incidents are many and occur far too often. Even if the material which is revealed is not particularly intimate, if it is information about a patient it should be protected.

social situations

Social situations present special problems. Physicians have to learn how to handle queries from a friend or a neighbor: "I hear John Peabody is in the hospital. How is he doing?" The physician soon learns, even though the inquiry may be friendly, to be extremely cautious about what he says. He has learned that by the time his comment passes through several hands it may be quite different from the one he actually expressed. "I don't know yet," he may reply. Or, "I can't tell you much. I'm not his doctor."

A nurse's aide from a small rural community said:

I used to get angry when some old busybody would come bustling up to me and say sweet-voiced, "Dearie, do tell me about Martha Burns. I hear she's got cancer."

I would snap back at her, "Why don't you ask her?" But now I like to play it a different way. I say, "Is that so?" and look at her real dumblike. "You must know something I don't know." And then I walk away.

I guess there are some people who don't have anything else to do but mind their neighbor's business. I don't waste a lot of steam anymore. I just think "that's the way they are, poor souls." And I try to keep out of their way. . . .

A nurse said:

You don't know when people ask about a patient what is real concern and what is just prying. I think most people don't mean any harm. But you can't risk a comment which seems harmless but might not be if you knew all the circumstances. I used to think it was better to make some noncommittal statement than just bluntly say I couldn't discuss the patient. I think I didn't want people to get angry with me. But now I just say, "Maybe you'd better talk to the doctor about that." I am careful about what I say to relatives, too, unless the doctor tells me to talk with them. Sometimes a relative will go around saying, "Well, the nurse said . . ." and maybe I didn't. She may have misunderstood me. Patients and their families don't always hear everything that is said to them.

special kinds of patients

Young women who are suspected of having entered the hospital to have an abortion or deliver an illegitimate child or patients thought to have some mental illness are objects of particular curiosity. The personnel on such wards must exercise unusual precautions in order to protect their patients and this means *all* personnel. Care must be taken in handling telephone inquiries or admitting strangers to the wards. There have been instances when a disturbed person, having somehow learned of an infant born out of wedlock, has tried to gain access to the ward to persuade the mother to give him the child. Infants have been kidnapped from the nursery of a hospital.

The health worker must take special care when he is away from the institution to avoid comments which might reveal information about patients. A grocer once said to the social worker on the psychiatric ward, "I see you have an amnesia victim on your ward."

"Do we?"

"Sure, it was in the newspapers. Most of those amnesia cases are phonies, anyway. I'll bet she'll come around after a few shock treatments."

The social worker would have liked to defend her patient, but she smiled sweetly and said, "Are you sure those sweetbreads are fresh?"

"Fresh! Of course, they are fresh. . . ."

As she left the store, the social worker said to her companion, "Everyone, but everyone, knows how to treat mental illness, even the corner grocer. And it wouldn't do a damn bit of good to try to tell him he's wrong. He knows. . . ."

the relative trap

Sometimes a health worker may be related to a patient. This can create real problems for him. He may get a great deal of pressure from other family members to divulge information. He may be curious himself about what is wrong with his relative. Just as a physician does not attempt to treat a member of his family who is ill, the health worker should not in most instances care for his relatives. Individual circumstances may create exceptions to this, but the decision should be made by his superior, not by the health worker himself. He should avoid reading the patient's chart, if he is related to him, unless he has permission to do so.

the medical chart

There is no other document on humans which contains so much intimate material as the medical chart and has the potential for so much help or harm. The staff who handle the information in a professional and responsible manner find it invaluable in caring for the sick. But not all personnel, even though they are authorized to read it, know how to handle the chart in such a way as neither to upset or to hurt the patient. Sometimes these are inexperienced people, students, perhaps, who have yet to learn. But sometimes, even with training, they may be insensitive to the feelings of patients. The seminary student in the first chapter was not only inexperienced but apparently unaware of how the patient felt at learning that he knew the nature of the surgery she was to have. Had he said, "I understand you are going to have surgery in a little while," this might have been acceptable to her, but to say bluntly, "I hear you are going to have a hysterectomy" was a violation of her privacy.

There is no way of knowing how often this kind of assault is committed upon a patient's very personal and intimate life. In the last chapter reading the medical chart was given as one of the ways to gain some knowledge of the patient. But the health worker can use this means only if he is authorized to read it. If he is not authorized to do so, he must learn to know his patients by some of the other methods discussed in the preceding chapter.

In most places the medical chart is carefully guarded, but in the best of institutions, human error may cause information to fall into the wrong hands. A student or staff person may leave a chart lying on a table. A volunteer worker wheeling a patient from one place to another must also take the chart with her and sometimes she lays it in the patient's lap while she maneuvers doors and elevators. If she should be called away, what patient can resist reading his chart? He is the one person who in most institutions is never allowed to read it.

A nurse observed a patient one day absorbed in his chart while waiting in one of the clinics. Someone had carelessly left it lying on the desk within reach of the patient. She walked over and took the chart from the patient, smiled at his look of chagrin, patted his shoulder, and walked away without saying a word.

In another instance, a young woman posing as a social worker asked for and received the chart of an infant available for adoption. The clerk had failed to ask for identification. It was later discovered that this woman had applied to a social agency for the adoption of this particular infant. Fortunately, the medical chart contained little information.

There are different legal opinions in various states as to whether a medical chart can be subpoenaed in insurance claims, compensation cases, or divorce cases. The health workers, responsible for the records, need to know the legal rulings of their particular state so they can protect the chart. Sometimes in cases where there is sensational material, the writing in the chart may be written in such a cryptic style that only the professional staff can identify it. In some instances, a second file is kept of extremely confidential material. Such devices as these are not the most satisfactory but they are intended to protect the patient and the institution.

inquisitive or unscrupulous people

A patient in a private room was lying with his eyes closed. He heard footsteps beside his bed and the voices of two women. One said: "This must be one of the boys in that highway accident." "He don't look too good, does he?" the other woman said.

The patient opened his eyes and they backed away still staring. "They didn't even apologize," the patient later told his family.

Unscrupulous individuals such as newspaper reporters or insurance adjusters sometimes gain access to a patient's room without having authorization. Not all reporters or insurance adjusters are like this, but there are some. The patient may make a statement or sign papers of release when he is hardly aware of what he is doing. Because the health worker sees more of the patient than the professional staff, he may be the first to be aware of what is happening.

protection from visitors

Some patients have strong feelings about having anyone but their family visit them when they are sick. Others cannot bear to be alone and want someone with them all the time. Others use their illness as a social affair and would like to have their room full of people day and night. This attitude about visitors often depends upon the personality of the patient and the nature of his illness.

Sometimes having visitors is a cultural affair. In some areas of the country, when a person becomes ill, all his relatives and friends gather around his bedside and remain until he is recovering or until he dies. In one large hospital a few years ago, the administrator came to work one morning and found all the chairs and lounges in the waiting room filled with sleeping people covered with blankets and with pillows under their heads.

"What has happened?" he asked thinking that there must have been some kind of disaster.

He found out that all the sleeping people were friends or relatives of an elderly patient who was critically ill. It was not easy to dissuade the family from using the waiting room as a dormitory. When the waiting room was repossessed, some of the family moved upstairs into the patient's room and others waited in the hall outside. This created problems for the staff in their efforts to care for the patient and it disturbed other patients. The administrator found it was not easy to try to change deeply rooted customs.

right to withhold information

Protection of the patient's right to withhold information is not always recognized as a responsibility of the health personnel. In the admitting office questions as to marital status may be embarrassing to the unwed mother who has brought her child to the clinic. Sometimes she may give a fictitious name for a husband. Another unwed mother may state her situation coldly and without emotion. The inexperienced or insensitive may think her "a shameless and brazen hussy." The skilled interviewer, however, learns to withhold judgment. She has learned that some of the most belligerent patients are the ones who "do all their crying inside."

Withholding of information about finances creates other problems. The admissions clerk must protect the institution but even if she suspects some discrepancy in the patient's statement, she will do better to listen politely and take her questions to her supervisor. Most patients are not dishonest, but at the time they are interviewed by the admissions desk they are under great stress, worrying about what may be wrong with them, what may need to be done, and what it all will cost. If they sense that the admissions clerk is concerned about helping them understand the admissions procedures, that she is not there "to turn them upside down and shake out the loose change," most patients will relax and try to give all the necessary information.

The following incident presents an example of a patient withholding information and describes the manner in which it was handled. This event occurred in a seminar on the psychiatric ward.

Only the chief social worker and the medical students attended the conference which was led by the staff psychiatrist. The patient's history had been presented by the student and then the patient was brought in for a brief interview. This interview was usually handled by the psychiatrist.

The patient was a middle-aged woman who had lived a life of great deprivation and tragedy. The staff psychiatrist was careful to ask only general, nontraumatic questions.

One of the medical students, however, interrupted to say triumphantly, "you were pregnant when you were married, weren't you?"

The patient did not reply, but looked at him with such anger that it filled the room. The psychiatrist broke the silence by saying gently, "You have been very helpful, but I wonder if you could describe the headaches you have been having, once again. I want to be certain I understand exactly how they affect you."

After a few more questions of a general nature, he stood and escorted the woman to the door. Thanking her, he patted her reassuringly on the back and dismissed her. Then he turned and walked back to the table and sat down again.

For a long while he just looked at the medical student; then he said in icy tones, "Don't ever again ask a patient that kind of question in that kind of way even if you are alone with her."

"But according to the chart . . ." the student began.

"When the patient gave the dates of her marriage and the birth of her first child she told you in the only way she could what had happened. She didn't lie. She could have. That she did not speak more frankly tells us that this experience is something she finds difficult to discuss. She has a right to determine when and to whom she will talk. All patients have this right and we must respect it."

Sometimes patients withhold information which may have serious implications for their health; knowledge about previous illnesses or allergies to certain drugs are example of this. In such cases, sometimes the patient may have to be protected from himself. Usually, if he has a good relationship with his physician he will not withhold anything. There are exceptions to this.

One patient was given a prescription for phenobarbital but did not take it. Her physician, who knew her very well, asked, "What are you afraid of, Martha?" As much as she liked and trusted him, she could not bring herself to tell him the reason. Her sister-in-law, who was with her, later said that Martha was afraid to take the drug because it was habit forming and she thought too that it was only given to epileptics. The sister-in-law didn't speak up earlier because she felt it wasn't her place to say anything. Perhaps it was—perhaps it wasn't. One can argue both ways.

Usually in such situations, the physician eventually learns the reason and helps the patient understand why she must take the medicine. Seldom is knowledge relating to a patient's illness the responsibility of the health worker, but there are exceptions to this. An example is the diabetic patient on a very strict diet who has friends smuggle candy into his room for him. Perhaps neither the patient nor his friends realize how dangerous this could be, or perhaps the patient doesn't care. Whatever the reason for his behavior, if the health worker becomes aware of this situation, he should not attempt to handle the problem himself, but report it to the nurse or the physician in charge of the case.

right to refuse medical treatment

It is often difficult for the staff, professional and nonprofessional, to accept the right of the patient to make his own decision about the kind of medical care he will accept. A physician makes a recommendation that a patient have surgery, for example. This recommendation is based upon examinations and laboratory tests and is in the best interest of the patient. The patient, however, may have many reasons for refusing to approve the physician's findings. The young woman who "did not want to be deformed"[2] illustrates this. Had the young resident in that case been more experienced and had better rapport with his patient, he might have been able to help her get over her fears, but again he might not have been successful. In such an instance, the patient's decision must be respected. It is hoped it will be accepted graciously and sympathetically, in such a manner that should the patient later change her mind she can return without "losing face."

In some cases of terminal illnesses the patient or his family may request that life not be prolonged by blood transfusions or other means. This is a controversial area both within the health field and without, but the patient's right to decide must be protected.

In several states, abortion laws have been liberalized to conform with the recent Supreme Court decision. However, this ruling has not resolved the emotional reactions of its opponents. This is a complicated issue, involving religious, social, legal, medical, and personal problems. The decision in these two instances, that of the terminally ill patient or the pregnant woman, must be determined by the physician and the family, or the physician and the patient.

protection from the health worker

Sometimes the patient is most in need of protection from the health worker. Excluding the incidents of physical abuse and neglect, and considering only such situations as the ones in the preceding paragraph, let us consider the importance of the health worker's behavior. At all times he must be careful to protect the patient from his own opinions and emotions whether he is in agreement or disagreement with the decision which has been reached. This requires no small amount of self-discipline.

[2]Chap 1.

An example illustrating this kind of problem is reported by a social worker in a large city hospital.

It so happened that we had five unwed mothers on the maternity ward at the same time. As I always did, I talked with all the young women about the plans they wished to make for their babies. I had several interviews with each of them before their babies were born. I also planned to interview them again after the birth of the babies in order to be as certain as possible that whatever decision they had made, it was the one they were most comfortable with. Every one of these situations is loaded with emotion and there is hurt for the young woman no matter what she decides.

Three of the young women decided prior to giving birth to relinquish their babies and all had good reasons for doing so. They signed the papers. After that, I am sorry to say I got very busy—no excuse, really—and did not return to the ward for a couple of days. The head nurse called me.

"I think you had better get up here. I am not sure just what is happening, but the three girls who relinquished their babies are all upset. One is crying."

I went right up and talked with each one of them separately. They were upset. They were tearful, angry at me for letting them sign the papers. They wanted to keep their babies now and they wanted to leave the hospital as soon as possible.

Not immediately, but eventually, I learned that one of the attendants on the maternity ward, a deeply religious woman, had approached each of the three young women and scolded them for the sin that they had committed in having become pregnant out of wedlock. Furthermore, she told them they would commit a double sin if they gave up the babies when they were born. The babies were "God's punishment" for the wicked life they had led and the cross they had to bear.

Older, more sophisticated women might not have re-

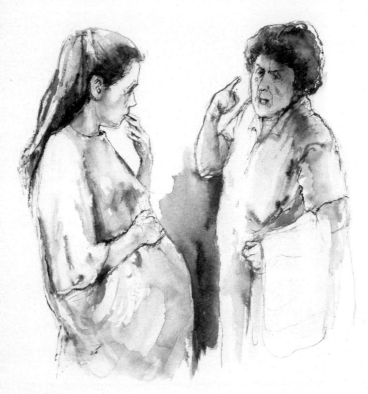

FIGURE 5

"One of the attendants on the maternity ward, a deeply religious woman, had approached each of the three young women and scolded her for the sin that she had committed in having become pregnant out of wedlock."

sponded as these girls did, but they were all quite young. Two had come from farm homes and one from a small town. None had had much experience.

I spent quite a bit of time with them, and made arrangements to follow them when they returned to their families. No, I didn't put any pressure on them to give up their babies. When people are very upset it's no time for them to

*make a decision about anything as important as giving up
a baby. Eventually two of the girls did elect to relinquish
their babies. The third girl kept hers. Her family did not
want the child, and I could see many problems ahead for
the baby and the girl, but it was her decision. All I could
do was keep the door open.*

*The nurse talked with the attendant, who saw nothing
wrong in her behavior, so strong were her convictions. She
was not dismissed. She had a right to her beliefs, but not
the right to impose them on other people. She was transferred to another department.*

SUMMARY: Protection of the patient can be a highly sensitive area—and there will be many times when the health
worker is helpless, because of his position or the rules of the
institution, to do anything, but he must be careful that he does
not use this as an excuse to do nothing. "It wasn't my
responsibility," or "It happens all the time. What can I do?" To
do nothing when a patient needs protection is bad for the
patient, but it is also a destructive experience for the health
worker. If nothing else let him be certain that he protects the
patient from his own acts of carelessness and irresponsibility.

If the health worker maintains as his base of operation the
patient's welfare, rather than institutional rules or job assignments, he may find there are many ways he can protect a
patient or make his stay in the institution less traumatic. An
example of the wrong way to care for a patient is the following
incident:

*An elderly man was admitted to the surgical ward as an
emergency. He had driven some two hundred miles to
reach the hospital. Not planning to stay, he had left his
car unlocked in the parking lot. Once admitted to the ward
he fretted over his car, and finally a request was sent
down to the social service department. The social worker
assigned to his care ignored several calls from the ward
about the car. When his supervisor asked him why he*

hadn't taken care of this matter, he replied haughtily "My
responsibility for a patient ends at the hospital door."
Technically he was right, but by every other measure he
was wrong. Going out to the parking lot to lock up a patient's
car was an item not listed in any job description, yet it was
something that needed to be done. And done quickly, if the
old man's anxiety was to be relieved.

There are many such examples, and often the health
worker's imagination and ingenuity will be under great pressure. He may also find that this is an area in which he will
receive few thanks. If he is told to ask a patient's visitors to
leave, because the visiting hours are over or because the
patient is tired, both the visitors and the patient may be angry
with him. If he feels he is not authorized to take responsibility
for direct action, he does have the responsibility to report to
his superior any occurrences which might be harmful to the
patient. Here again, he may meet with a rebuff. The superior
may be too busy to investigate, or may not think it important.
Sometimes the health worker is made to feel he is being
overzealous.

After reading the examples in this chapter, the health
worker may take small comfort from the fact that not only he
but the professional commits many "acts of omission." In this
area professionals as well as health workers have had little
training and usually learn at the expense of the patient.

ASSIGNMENT: As you go about your daily routine, take note
of incidents involving patient protection. Hopefully, you will
observe some positive examples as well as negative ones. Give
some thought to the probable effect upon the patient of these
occurrences, positive and negative.

"Take it easy, for a while. . . ."

"I don't want to be a superspy."

"Why didn't you come to me earlier?"

"Mother just couldn't take it."

"If you don't eat your meat, you can't have any dessert."

"You poor little thing."

"He will outgrow this, won't he?"

"There is nothing wrong with my mind."

". . . I don't want to be a baby factory."

". . . one final courtesy. . . ."

6 special kinds of patients

"All patients are special," said the author, firmly.
"Yes, I know," replied the health worker, hastily. "I was
just thinking, though, are there particular things to look
out for with certain kinds of patients?"
"I am not sure," the author said thoughtfully, "that we will
see any significant differences in the way patients should
be cared for by putting them into categories. However,
such an arrangement might serve to reemphasize patient
needs and more clearly define the role of the health
worker. Suppose we try it. . . ."

the human variable

All patients are special and to try to put them into categories by generalizations such as "All paraplegics respond in such and such a manner," or "All cardiac patients have these characteristics" would be misleading. Every patient is a particular kind of person and illness or injury only reinforces or emphasizes the personality characteristics he already has. True, in some illnesses there may be personality changes, in patients with certain kinds of head injuries, for example. It is also true, as we have learned, that patients go through a series of reactions to their illness or injury, but as we have also discovered there are as many variations in these responses as there are people to express them. We should, however, be able to make some general observations if we remember the "human variable."

cardiac patients

A few years ago a research team made a follow-up study of some twenty-five children who had received corrective heart surgery some ten years previously. The surgery performed at one of the research institutes in the Northwest had been considered successful. The children, all very young, were discharged after a few clinic visits and none of them had been seen since then.

The research team, after some difficulty, was able to locate most of the children and their families. The children, with few exceptions, seemed to have had no serious medical problems since their surgery. However, the interviewers were not prepared for the emotional responses of both parents and children—nor did they know how to handle such reactions. The parent, usually the mother, was found in a number of the cases to be exceedingly anxious and fearful. "I have tried to do what the doctors told me to do," was a common remark. Questioned as to exactly what the physicians had instructed them to do at the time the children were discharged, the mothers replied with vague statements such as, "He said not to let Tina try to do too much," "Be sure Johnny gets plenty of rest." When asked how long the doctors had told them such instructions should be carried out, the mothers did not know. To try to recall the exact wording of the physician's orders after ten years was impossible. What the physicians had said, or how much of the instructions given were understood and comprehended by the parents, will never be known.

It was the impression, however, of the research staff that the parents had continued the protective role they had assumed prior to surgery when the children were young and ill. At that time such a role might have been appropriate, and perhaps it was also necessary for a while after surgery. The children of such parents had developed over the years a passive semi-invalid role. Not surprisingly, the research team found that the children's attendance at school was irregular and that they did not participate in many teen-age activities. In general, their social adjustment seemed poor. The research team recognized that factors other than the heart surgery might have influenced the children's poor socialization, but their illness appeared to have had a profound influence upon them.

There was little the research team could do other than recommend that the children be returned to the institute for a current evaluation of their physical condition, and they also advised referral of both parent and child to a counseling service. Such counseling probably was ten years too late, because by then both parents and children had a fixed pattern of behavior.

Cardiac patients and their families are anxious people, although one must remember that anxiety accompanies all illnesses. In the cardiac, though, it would seem especially important that there be good and clear communication between the physician and his patient. The physican may say to a cardiac, "Take it easy for a while, John" and both John and his family hear only the "Take it easy," not the "for a while." Not infrequently the physician is later heard to remark, "I told John to take it easy for a while and he hasn't done a lick of work since then." Who is at fault in such cases, the patient or the physician? Both, perhaps. The physician should know that he must spell out very carefully and more than once the instructions for his patient. Often these instructions need to be repeated by his nurse or some other staff person.

At the time a patient and his family are first told the nature of the illness they are often in a state of shock. They literally do not hear all the physician is saying to them. "They hear only what they want to hear," the physician may counter, and sometimes this seems to be true. A dependent person may interpret the words "Take it easy, John" as permission to give up his lifelong struggle to be independent and self-sustaining. To another patient the same words may be a terrible threat. He sees the command "Take it easy" as an order to give up the things from which he derives the greatest satisfaction, his work, his play, and he may react by driving himself to do more and more as if to prove the physician is wrong. This points up the necessity of the physician's knowing his patient very well before making any recommendation.

And the families. Their interpretations of the physician's instructions may also be made in the light of their own needs. If a wife or mother is dominant and aggressive she may interpret the physician's directions to mean that she take over and manage the husband and his affairs or that she continue to control the life of her child. Remember, however, not all wives or mothers (or husbands or fathers) do this even though they may be aggressive. One needs to know the individual situation. Each one is different.

A wife who has a great dependence on her husband may be so frightened at the threat of his illness that she becomes more helpless and dependent, and demands more of the patient than he is physically able to give.

If the wife, however, can manage her own feelings appropriately, she can do much to help her husband make a good recovery or make a satisfactory adjustment to his illness. In quiet, unobtrusive ways, she can limit the patient's activity—yet at the same time encourage him to gradually become more active. This means the wife must have a good understanding of her husband's condition. She must also know how to interpret the physician's recommendations. Involvement of the family in the treatment plan is important. The physician needs to know not only his patient, but his patient's family.

"All right! All right!" the health worker says impatiently.
"You have talked about what a cardiac condition means to the family and what the physician should do, but what about me? What do I do?"
"Let's talk about that," the author responds, "but first tell

me, have you ever noticed how much more relaxed the patient often is and how much more freely he speaks when the professionals aren't around, when only health workers are present?"

"I'll buy that, if you mean the patients talk and act as if we weren't there. Sometimes, the way they sound off, I think we must be invisible."

"I view such behavior in a slightly different way," said the author, smiling a little. "I think patients feel more comfortable with health workers. You don't threaten them as much. The patient can let down his guard and be himself."

"Well," the health worker said, "I don't know about that." He was pleased, however.

"If my impressions are correct, health workers are in a position to know the patient much better than the doctor or other professionals can. Take the patient who was terrified at learning he had a heart condition. It is very likely that he showed the doctor none of his fear, but said 'Yes doctor, I understand. Thank you.' When he walked out of the doctor's office and thought no one was observing him, he may well have sworn, 'That damn doctor! What does he know?' and marched angrily down the hall. Again, this same patient may have held himself together, head erect, shoulders back, a smile on his face, until the door of the doctor's office closed behind him, and then his shoulders may have sagged. He looked straight ahead not seeing anyone or anything. His hands shook as he pulled out a cigarette. All this behavior is obviously quite different from the manner he displayed in the doctor's office.

"Let us take this example one step further," continued the author. "Who is the person most likely to see the patient after he leaves the doctor's office? The health worker. What does he do if he observes the patient acting strangely?"

"I suppose he should try to get hold of the nurse."

"That would be good. If he knew the doctor well he might

speak to him. 'I don't know what you said to that patient, doc, but he acted kind of strange after he left your office. I was a little worried about him.'"
The health worker had a peculiar look on his face.
"I don't want to be a superspy," he said uneasily.
The author was quite serious. "You are a part of the health care staff. If you have knowledge of a patient which indicates he is anxious or in any way upset, you have a responsibility to put that information into the hands of someone who can use it. Someone who can utilize your knowledge to better understand the patient and help him more effectively."
The health worker sighed. "You win. But," he added with some of his old aggressiveness, "it seems to me that whatever we talk about, it turns out to be my responsibility."
"Oh, we will still leave a few of the responsibilities for patient care to the professionals," replied the author dryly.
"We have," she continued, "spent considerable time on the cardiac, but many of the things we have discussed can also apply to other kinds of patients. Let us now look at the cancer patient."

cancer patients

The word "cancer" frightens people. It may be that this is the reason some patients delay seeking medical advice after they discover symptoms. Fear may be expressed in different ways. "I am afraid I will hear something I don't want to hear." Others have a fatalistic attitude: "I'm going to die anyway. Why bother!" Another form of fear is denial: "If I wait long enough the symptoms will go away." There are other patients who hesitate to visit their doctor because "he will think I am just imagining all this." Sensible responses? No, but people who are afraid are neither sensible or rational beings.

A visit to the doctor's office is not always reassuring.

Should he ask, "Why didn't you come to me earlier?" the patient interprets this to mean, "I've come too late. I am going to die." Even if the doctor senses the patient's alarm and tries to reassure him, the patient is still anxious. "He just didn't want to scare me," the patient may say to his family. Another fear of patients, expressed or unexpressed, is fear of pain. The wise physician anticipates this concern and carefully explains to the patient and his family what can be expected and what can be done about it.

When the diagnosis is cancer, families and friends do not always help. One patient said:

When I told my family that the doctor said I had cancer and would require surgery, they were upset, but they tried to say the right things, like it was to be only minor surgery, and lots of people had it and had no further trouble. All of which is true enough, but their voices gave them away and also the look in their eyes. They made me feel as if I were dead and buried and they were about to begin dividing up my belongings.

They meant all right. They're good people, but they were scared. I was too. We ... well ... we just didn't know how to communicate. It took a while before any of us could act naturally.

There often seems to be reluctance to tell a patient the diagnosis. One doctor said, "Some of my patients would go to pieces if I mentioned the word "cancer" to them. I don't deceive them, but I talk about what needs to be done and I encourage them to ask questions. Should they ask me point blank if they have cancer, I tell them." Another physician speaks emphatically: "I never lie to my patients. They know that and they trust me. Yes, some take it harder than others, but you know I don't think you ever fool a patient. They know what's wrong." Still a third physician remarked quietly, "Doctors are human, you know. It is not easy to have to give bad news to a patient, especially if you have known them and their family for a long time." Families sometimes request that the patient not be told. "Mother just couldn't take it." "I want my wife to be happy as long as she can." Families are often protecting themselves by such appeals. The patient, even a frightened patient, shows remarkable fortitude when he knows what is wrong. Usually he gets along better if the diagnosis is given to him. However, the decision as to whether he should be told is most often made by the patient's physician.

Families and friends and health care staff can handle acute illnesses or emergencies better than they can handle illnesses which drag out for a long period of time. At first everyone rallies around, eager to help, but as time goes on, friends drift away and families become restless and uncomfortable. Patients are acutely aware of the change in attitude.

One of them described her reactions:

I was one of the fortunate ones. Some years ago I had a diagnosis of cancer. I was operated on and had some plastic surgery. It was several months before I could go back to work part-time, but it was a good thing I did go. I had reached the point where I couldn't stand my family and I am sure they felt the same way about me.

At first my family and my friends crowded around and tried to do everything they could, but after a while my friends began to come around less often and my family seemed bored. I don't think my family ever wished me dead but they acted as if my illness were a nuisance. I felt the same way about it myself.

I could not but think of an old woman I used to know who lived back in the hills. She had many tragedies in her life. After one of them, I said, "You must be feeling very badly."

"No," she replied, "I am jest all dreened out of feeling."

I think my friends, my family, and I, too, reached the point where we were "all dreened out of feeling."

I was glad, believe me, to get back to work where people knew nothing of my illness and where I could begin to forget it, myself. . . ."

"Well," said the health worker, "we're back to the bit about the understanding doctor and the understanding family."
"And the understanding health worker," replied the author.

In cases where there is cancer or cancer is suspected, families and patients are anxious. They are supersensitive to the reactions of all the people around them. They are constantly looking for clues which may reveal the things they fear the doctor has not told them.

In such cases as these the role of the health worker, always important, assumes special significance, because the patient and even his family may try to get information from him they cannot get or dare not ask of the physician. A seemingly innocent question, "Do you see many patients like me?" or a more loaded question, "I know you see a lot of patients like me. What do you think my chances are?" may take the health worker by surprise. Unless he thinks quickly and

"Keeps his cool," interrupts the health worker.

"Right. Keeping your cool is most important. A slight hesitation, a too-glib response may be interpreted by the patient as 'he's keeping something from me, too. He knows I'm not going to make it.'" The author stopped and then asked, "How would you answer such questions. Let's take the first one." The health worker grimaced. "It would depend on what I was supposed to be doing."

"That's correct. Suppose you are an attendant."

"Well, I might say, 'Oh, I see all kinds of patients.' No, that's no good. That's the glib kind of answer, isn't it? How about just saying, 'What do you mean?'"

"Not a bad answer, but what if the patient then says, 'Oh, you know what I mean. People who have the same thing I do.'"

The health worker thought about this question. "I guess I'd say, 'I'm afraid you're talking to the wrong person because I don't know much about such things.'"

"Is that all you would say? Think! Why did the patient ask these questions?"

"He was scared."

"Well, what do you do about his fear?"

"I'm not sure," the health worker said slowly. "How about, 'if you are worried, maybe you ought to talk to someone who could help you.'"

The author nodded approvingly. "The patient then may say, 'No one will tell me a thing.'"

"Have you tried talking to your doctor?"

"He's just like everyone else. He won't tell me a thing."

"Does he know you are worried?"

"Hell, he ought to."

"Maybe you have to spell it out for him. . . ."

The author and the health worker looked at each other and laughed. "Do you know what we have been doing?" the author asked. "We've been role playing."

"Is that what you call it? I'd call it play acting."

"The same thing. It's one method we use in teaching human behavior. To get back to our patient. You would use some of the same kind of responses for the second question. You would also want to be sure to let the doctor or the nurse know the patient was worried and asking such questions. The patient might not be able to bring himself to speak to his doctor."

"Remember," the author continued, "in the cases where the patient has cancer, just as with the cardiac patients, the health worker may be the first member of the health care staff to sense the patient's fear and discouragement, or to be aware of the family's impatience and in some instances to realize that they are drifting away from the patient. The way you treat the patient, your attitude, may influence the family's behavior."

stroke and spinal cord injuries

Without going into the medical aspects of strokes and spinal cord injuries, it can be said these are two of the most common causes for paralysis, whether the paralysis is permanent or only temporary. The shock to the family and the patient is great. The suddenness of the trauma is one reason for the reaction of both family and patient. For example one day the patient is a competent and successful business man and perhaps overnight he lies in bed completely helpless, unable to move, incontinent, perhaps unable to speak or unconscious. Consider an active, confident, outgoing teen-ager who has an automobile accident and overnight he, too, lies helpless and immobilized, with all the bright hopes he and his family had for his future seemingly shattered. In addition to the suddenness of the incapacity another factor which adds to the family's distress and the patient's, if he is aware of what is going on, is that often the physician cannot always immediately evaluate the damage and make any prediction as to how much recovery can be expected.

Therefore, the first few weeks are a time of great tension for the family and for the patient, again if he is aware of what is going on. Both react. The family alternately pleads and demands that the doctor give them some idea of what to expect—what the outcome of the illness or injury will be. The patient may not voice his concern as vehemently as the family, but he has it, nonetheless. Remember the discussion in Chapter 3 of the different emotional stages the patient goes through in adjusting to trauma. The first stage, fear or anxiety, is that which seems to occur in most patients in the first few weeks immediately following the illness or injury.

The stroke patient, depending upon which part of the brain is damaged, may show behavior quite different from that his family has come to expect from him. He may expose himself, push his food onto the floor, hold a pill under his tongue and not swallow it. He may cry. One case was that of a sweet little old lady who had gone to church every Sunday of her life. After a stroke she used the most indescribable language and left her family and the minister in a state of shock.

It is difficult for the family to understand and accept the fact that the patient is not responsible for his actions. When he does something particularly childish, such as throwing his food on the floor, the family often scolds him. Strange as it may seem, they sometimes get angry with him if he continues to "misbehave." The family's anger is often based on fear. Their world as they have known it, their relationship with the patient from whom they have come to expect rational behavior, seems destroyed.

Even though the doctor and the nurse may say repeatedly that the patient cannot help the things he does, the family seems not able to hear them. In such instances the patient has to have protection from his family. If he has any understanding of what is going on around him, his family's reactions may add one more stress to the many he is attempting to adjust to. If he is only partially able to comprehend what is happening he may sense his family's anger from the tone of their voice.

Because of the emotional involvement of the families, stroke patients often do better in a nursing home where the staff has experience in knowing how to care for them. To treat a stroke patient as a child when he does something childish does no good. The experienced health workers in nursing homes treat childish behavior by ignoring it. They neither cajole nor threaten "if you don't eat your meat you can't have any dessert." They praise the patient and pay him little attentions but accept the fact that his behavior will not change. In most stroke patients, while they may regain some of their motor facilities, there is usually little improvement in their intellectual functioning. It is also well to keep in mind that the same condition that caused the initial stroke is causing some degeneration elsewhere in the brain. Often other strokes will occur—each causing more brain damage. This is another reason why a nursing home may be the best solution. These are difficult patients to care for. Even if the family is understanding, few homes are equipped to provide the proper equipment and care. On the other hand, there is no solution other than the home, however poorly equipped it is, whatever the attitude of the family, if there is not money enough to pay for the nursing home. A tragic dilemma for both family and patient.

Spinal cord injuries may result in partial or total paralysis. These injuries are not reversible. Unless there is some kind of head injury in addition to the damage to the spinal cord there is no impairment of intellect. Many of these injuries are the result of automobile accidents and many of the victims are adolescents. This kind of injury is a tragedy for anyone, but to a young and energetic boy or girl it must seem the end of the world, and it is the end of involvement in many activities valued by the young.

Rehabilitation for these patients can be difficult. Alternately rebellious and deeply discouraged, it is not easy to get the patient's cooperation in the hours, days, and months of physical therapy, bladder control and training in self-maintenance. It is often difficult to maintain their interest in vocational training. The patience of the staff and family is often under severe strain. A nurse comments:

I remember one day I saw three boys in wheelchairs racing down the hall of the hospital. They managed the chairs quite skillfully and had great fun wheeling as close to a passerby as they could without touching him. Anyone hearing only their laughter and jokes, and not seeing the wheelchairs, would have thought them typical teen-agers, a little obnoxious, but obviously having a good time.

No one reprimanded them for their behavior. I smiled at them remembering all they had been through and thinking of some of the more severely injured patients on the ward who would never be able to sit in a wheelchair. As I watched them I thought of the task someone would have of helping these boys through an abnormal adolescence and guiding them into maturity. Families couldn't do it by themselves.

I recalled a man I saw at the grocery store the other day. A middle-aged man, he too was in a wheelchair. He was alone. He went about picking up groceries from the shelves paying attention to no one. I wondered what he would do if he wanted something from an upper shelf but apparently he knew what he wanted and had no intention of asking anyone for help. He may have been too independent. I would like to have known more about him. . . .

Families and staff, too, have difficulty in maintaining discipline with young patients who have severe injuries. Families especially, are inclined to be too indulgent and too ready to do things for the patient rather than trying to help him grow up and to do as much as possible for himself. One of the reasons for keeping such patients in a rehabilitation unit for a long time is to give them as much training as possible in caring for themselves. Some of this families cannot do. Also the patients will take guidance from the health care staff more readily than from their parents.

"What do you think is the most important quality a health worker must have to care for this group of patients?" the author asked.

"Understanding?"

"That is important, understanding of patients, of families, and of one's self. I was thinking, however, of patience. It seems to me that is the most needed quality in dealing with the patients or families with all the adjustments both must make."

brain-damaged patients

Patients who are brain damaged may be crippled, have poor muscular control, and have difficulty in speaking. In some cases there is mental retardation. These symptoms of trauma are among the more common ones but there are many others. In some patients a combination of symptoms may be found. For example, the patient with poor muscular control may be retarded and speak with difficulty. However, the important thing for the health worker to understand is that in any of these symptoms there may be a *difference* in the amount of brain damage. For instance, one patient may have a hardly noticeable speech impairment, while another patient may have such difficulty in speaking it is hard to understand him. One patient may be only slightly retarded, while another patient may require custodial care. Too often, there is a tendency to classify brain-damaged patients as epileptics, spastics, or mentally retarded persons without recognition that each patient is different and that the amount of handicap is never the same in any two cases.

Brain damage indicates that some injury has occurred to the brain or that there is some degree of malfunction in that organ. For the purposes of this book it is not necessary to discuss the causes or other medical aspects of damage to the brain. They are complicated. However, if the health worker is employed in an institution, clinic, or school for the handicapped, where many of the patients will have this kind of handicap, he should have more knowledge if he is to perform effectively. There are many books and professional articles written about the brain-damaged patient, but the health worker should start by taking his questions to his superior.

When a baby is born with indications it is brain damaged (sometimes the symptoms may not be apparent until later) the physician has to decide when and how to tell the parents. If he waits too long, they may learn the tragic news from someone else.

"Yes," said the health worker, "I know a case like that. A nurse's aide in the nursery went to the mother's room to get the baby and take it back to the nursery. As she was carrying the baby out of the mother's room she said, "You poor little thing," and the mother heard her.

The health worker shook his head, "The nurse's aide didn't mean any harm. She was a kind woman. She just didn't think."

Telling the parents that their baby is handicapped is never

an easy task for the physician. He also has some emotional investment in the baby he has delivered. When he first tries to explain the nature of the brain damage to the parents, the physician often finds they are in shock and do not really hear him. Any discussion of the prognosis and future plans means little to the parents at this time. In their sorrow and disbelief, they may say, "I don't understand. He looks perfectly normal," or "He will outgrow this, won't he?" There is sometimes anger toward the physician. "Was this something that happened when you were delivering the baby," or "Couldn't you have done something to prevent this?"

Underneath, however, parents often blame themselves. If the baby was unwanted, if an unsuccessful abortion was attempted, if the father was unfaithful, these and many other reasons, logical or illogical, may cause a parent to condemn himself or his marriage partner. Sometimes, especially when the damage is severe, the parents may wish the child had never been born. This feeling, too, may never find expression.

The health worker must be cautioned, however. As was stated at the beginning of this chapter, broad generalizations cannot be made. It would be grossly inaccurate to say that all parents had such feelings as we have described. Every mother and father is a different kind of person. It is important that as the health worker observes the parents, the way they handle the baby, the things they say and do, he make some estimate of how they feel in order to give them, the parents, the kind of care they badly need. For example, if the mother has been told of her baby's disability while she is still in the hospital, she may need some extra "mothering." Nothing sloppy or sentimental, but gentle, unobtrusive acts of kindness. The health worker must not discuss feelings with the mother. This is not his role; nonetheless, the things he can and should do are just as important as the professionals' responsibilities.

Particularly in the early years of the child's life there are frequent contacts with members of the health care staff. The parents may go "shopping around" trying to find someone who will tell them their child is "perfectly normal," or that there is a new drug or some kind of surgery which will produce a cure. Often the health care staff gets impatient. "Can't they understand?" "Why do they take up everyone's time?" No one can *make* parents understand and accept such an unpleasant truth. They must be allowed to move, sometimes slowly, but at their own pace, toward realization and some kind of acceptance or resignation. These parents need much understanding and kindness. They are often difficult and demanding, quick to detect any sign of impatience, dislike, or aversion on the part of the health care staff.

Brain damage is irreversible. If the child is so severely handicapped that he requires institutional care, this too is something that parents may find difficult to face. The staff of institutions for the handicapped also have problems of adjustment. It is discouraging and demoralizing to have to work eight hours a day with a group of patients who will be able to show only limited improvement. The professionals can handle this problem by working only part-time in the institution, or by spending part of the day in research, writing, or teaching. The health workers, however, usually must spend the entire eight hours, day after day, with patients who require much care and who may be unattractive and difficult to like or to love.

"Some of the health workers I know don't seem to mind working with the handicapped," the health worker commented. "They seem to get satisfaction out of seeing that the patients are kept clean, fed, and cared for, and I have known some of them who got real involved, maybe too much so, and worried and fussed over the patients as if they were their own people."

"Yes, I know many such health workers and there's no place in health care where they are needed more. However, if a health worker in one of these institutions gets discouraged I hope he will look for some alternatives before he decides to leave his job. Some institutions allow the health worker to take time off for further schooling. In

other places, group meetings are arranged where the health workers can talk of their feelings and are encouraged to participate in plans for relieving the monotony of their daily tasks. Job rotation is also practiced in other places."

The role of the health worker in dealing with brain-damaged patients within and outside of institutions also requires much patience and courtesy. Families and many of the patients are unusually sensitive. There is resentment if the patient is stared at, laughed at, treated as a freak, or talked to as if he were a child, when he is an adult.

"There is nothing wrong with my mind," a cerebral palsied patient said sadly to his social worker. He was a wheelchair invalid with poor muscular control who spoke with great difficulty, grimacing, and slobbering. He had experienced many rebuffs.

"Brain-damaged patients can often come to some kind of terms with their handicap if they are given a chance," he said. "It is never easy but it can be done, if only people realize that inside we have the same kinds of feelings they have. . . ."

unwanted pregnancy

A number of years ago a psychiatrist was quoted as saying that there would be no neurotics if the only babies born were wanted babies. That is the kind of statement which looks good until you look more closely at it. Wanted babies! Sometimes babies are wanted for the wrong reasons. For example, a couple may wish to have a child in order to salvage a poor marriage. Another couple may want a child "because our parents want a grandchild."

The Supreme Court decision of 1973 on abortions brought to the surface many reactions based on religious, ethical, medical, and social grounds. There is and will be ferment for a long time before the subject is viewed with objectivity. Meanwhile health workers and professional members of the health care staff have had to reexamine their own feelings about abortion and learn how to manage them. In one hospital the physicians and nurses met informally for a series of discussions on how they were going to handle the subject. In another hospital a psychiatrist met with professionals and health workers on the obstetrical service to help them in defining their role and to teach them some ways in which they could learn to manage their feelings. Everyone has some opinion and some feeling about abortions—the health care staff is no exception. Whatever feelings they have, however, these must not in any way influence their treatment of patients.

The author stopped and said to the health worker, "I am not asking how you feel about abortions. That is your personal and private business. I am saying that the health worker who approves of abortions must keep his objectivity as much as if he disapproves. He must keep his focus on the fact that the woman seeking or having an abortion is a patient and must be treated with no more or no less concern and respect than other patients are treated."

The health worker sighed. "This is one of the roughest things I have come up against. You get it from all sides. Someone trying to get you to take a stand on abortions. Not only people in the institution, but outside people, when they find you work in a hospital. It is tough trying not to commit yourself."

"If it's hard for you, just remember it's far more difficult for the woman considering an abortion. One young woman wrote this letter to her counselor:

'I have made up my mind. I am going to have an abortion. It will do no good for you to preach anymore Hellfire and Damnation to me. I will carry my own private hell in my heart for the rest of my life.

'You said why didn't I go on and have the baby and if I didn't want it, I could give it up for adoption. There were a lot of couples, you told me, who wanted a baby very much, but who couldn't have one. Well I feel sorry for such people, but I don't want to be a baby factory. How do I know that the family who adopted my baby would love

him in the right kind of way? You can't guarantee that, nor can anyone else. I have seen some adoptive parents I wouldn't give a sick cat to.

'I am sorry to disappoint you. You meant well even though I sometimes felt you didn't try hard enough to help me sort out my feelings because you were so busy thinking of the baby I was going to have. But I guess it comes down to the fact that no one else can make the decision. I feel better now that I have decided what I will do.'"

The health worker frowned. "It doesn't sound as if that counselor was objective."

"No, it doesn't, but we can't be sure of that without knowing the whole story."

Even though the pregnancy is unwanted, the woman may decide to continue with it. If she is married she usually keeps the baby, but today many unwed mothers are also deciding to bring up their babies by themselves. Other mothers elect to relinquish the baby for adoption. Whatever decision the mother and father make when the baby is not wanted is not made without conflict—without some "private hell." If they seek counseling, and usually they need it, they should have the very best. Unfortunately when people are in need they are not always able to choose wisely.

Also, since anyone, regardless of training, experience, or motivation, can call himself a counselor, the woman who has an unwanted pregnancy is sometimes subjected to great pressures: to have an abortion or not to have one; to continue the pregnancy and keep the baby; or to place it for adoption. Many times these recommendations are not made in the best interests of the mother or child. It is not surprising that many women, in order to protect themselves from such pressures, shut themselves off from any kind of counseling, good or bad.

dying patients

If the health worker is interested in learning more about the dying patient there are a number of books and professional articles available. His role as a health worker, however, may not be as well defined as he would wish, in such material. He may have to obtain most of his knowledge in the performance of his assigned responsibilities. He will discover that before he can help others face death and dying he must be able to handle his own feelings. People often think they know how until confronted with an actual experience. Take for example the report of a young lawyer:

"I grew up in the West and I was nourished on stories of the early days when men met their fate bravely and died with their boots on. That was the way I wanted to die, I thought—standing erect, looking my enemy straight in the eye, asking no quarter and giving none. However, in law school, I had an experience which caused me to be less sure that was a good idea.

"One of our professors was a great teacher. His dry, sarcastic way of speaking made his lectures enjoyable and unforgettable. When he developed cancer he made no secret of it. He continued to keep to his regular schedule and for a while his illness wasn't noticeable. As time went on, however, he had days when he appeared quite ill, but he still delivered his lectures in a grim no nonsense manner which neither permitted nor invited sympathy. At first, I think all the students admired him very much for his bravery. After a while, though, as he grew more ill and began having great difficulty in finishing his lectures, our feelings began to change. At least they did for some of us.

"The class met in the late afternoon. When it was finished I got into the habit of making for the nearest bar. Some of my classmates followed me. We would talk about the professor, how much guts he had, and we would wonder whether we could do what he was doing. I don't think we ever put into words our wish that it was all over, but we would talk about the strain and wonder how long we could take it. 'What would we do if he dropped dead right in the classroom?' While we expressed concern for the professor, I think we were primarily preoccupied with our

own feelings. To sit and watch a man die a little each day was almost more than we could bear. Toward the end he was brought to the class in a wheelchair. Shortly afterwards, he entered the hospital and died soon after he was admitted. I heard he refused any treatment which might have prolonged his life.

"The memory of this experience has come back to me many times. I have tried to understand it. I think it must have been very important for the professor to have handled his illness in this way. I am sure it took great courage and determination, but it was very hard on his students, and I have often wondered how his behavior affected his family and his colleagues, who knew him more intimately than did his students. . . ."

The health worker considered this narrative with a frown. "That guy wouldn't have made a good health worker."

"With training," the author replied, "he might have been a very good health worker. When you started out very likely you had some of the same kinds of feelings. They are not uncommon."

The health worker ignored this last comment. He was grim. "Well, I don't like that guy. Not at all. The only thing he is thinking about is his own feelings. He would have liked for his professor to have done his dying off in a corner where no one would have seen him."

The author was patient but firm. "Now, stop and look at what you are doing. You have to get your feeling in balance. You are all the way over in the professor's corner. Remember you have had more experience than the law students in seeing dying patients. You have more understanding of how patients cope with dying. You have had people around you with more knowledge than you have to teach you how to help and understand what death means to a patient and his family. These law students apparently had no one to help them sort out their own feelings. Their conversations among themselves may only have reinforced their own anxieties. You must have seen families who had some of the same feelings the law students had. What about the family who can't bear to stay in the room with their dying relative—who rush in and rush out again after only a few minutes? Surely you have heard a family pleading with the doctor to keep a dying patient in the hospital "where he will be more comfortable," or "better taken care of" than at home.

The health worker looked very uncomfortable. "Well," he said, "well, oh, blast it, I guess I have been mainly concerned with the patient."

"I want you to keep your concern for patients, but families need your concern, too. "Why do you think families or the law students act as these did?"

"I guess they were afraid."

"Yes, afraid. Also, they didn't know what to do. Most people don't know how to act in the presence of a dying patient. They may have had youthful fantasies, as did the law student, of what they themselves would do when faced with their own death or that of someone near to them, but no one knows how he will act or even how he should act."

The health worker, however, must have some fairly clear concept of his role, because he will often be involved in some aspect of care for the dying patient and his family. He must remember that the family may need his services more than the patient. With both, he must be unobtrusive, and walk quietly but not tiptoe. He must be kind. He must be concerned but not with any show of emotion. He should avoid the thoughtless remarks often heard at such times. Never tell a dying patient, "Oh, you will feel better tomorrow," or say to a family, "I know just how you feel." No one knows how anyone else feels unless that person tells him. If the health worker doesn't know what to say it is best to remain silent.

Ask a family or the patient if there is anything they want or anyone they want to see. Never ask if they wish to see a clergyman. They will tell you if this is what they want. For some families and patients such a question would be an insult.

Remember in Chapter 2 the social worker's narrative of

her experience on the cancer ward?[1] Recall her comment that the patients were alone much of the time. The literature on the dying patient notes the reluctance of both professional staff and health worker to spend much time with this kind of patient. Rather than avoiding the dying patient the health worker should visit frequently—never leave him alone for too long. There may be nothing he needs, but the visit is one final courtesy which the dying patient deserves.

SUMMARY: Every patient is special. That must always be the emphasis for the health worker. Particular illnesses or injuries, however, may require of him specific qualities, such as patience in caring for stroke and spinal cord injuries or objectivity in dealing with the subject of abortion.

In each of these categories the discussion was limited to those aspects of the illness or injury which might best illustrate the role of the health worker. He should realize, however, that he is only at the beginning of learning, not only about these special categories of patients but about all patients.

ASSIGNMENT: Choose a patient you have known who belonged in one of the categories discussed in this chapter. Identify if possible the attitude in yourself you found most useful in caring for him or her.

[1]Chap. 2, the section on the dying patient.

"Where did *he* come from?"

". . . out from under a rock. . . ."

"As if we had time to provide special diets!"

"It would have been better if father could have told me himself."

"She needs to see you."

"Your people only come so they can laugh at you. . . ."

". . . I sound as if I were the patient."

"My husband whom I loved. . . ."

"It's the memories. . . ."

". . . this kid will *never* walk."

". . . as if he came from nowhere and would vanish into the unknown. . . ."

7 families: the worst problem

"I guess that's right. Families are the worst problem," the health worker said. "They get in the way and ask stupid questions. If I had anything to say about it. . . ."

"Yes, I know . . ." the author said dryly, "if you had your way relatives would never be allowed to set foot in the institution."

"Now, wait a minute. I didn't say that."

"But you thought it and most of us in the health field have felt that way. Why is it they are such a problem—the families of patients?"

"Well. . . ."

"Suppose we try to find out . . . there must be a reason."

importance of patient's background

"Where did he come from?" some member of the staff will ask, but the question is usually rhetorical, because actually there is little interest in who or what the patient was before he came to a health care facility. Sometimes there is an attitude of annoyance in the query, "Where did *he* come from?" as if "the patient had climbed up out of a sewer or out from under a rock somewhere."

In spite of talk of treating the "whole patient" he is still far too often seen as an illness or an injury. Appropriate techniques of a surgeon or physician are utilized. Nursing care is provided. Indeed, all the paraphernalia of modern medicine may be involved in his care. Only at a time of crisis where, for example, a blood transfusion is needed, surgery is required, the patient is placed on the critical list, or is ready for discharge is there a flurry of activity to locate relatives. Urgent phone calls go out from the hospital, memos are sent down to the social service department, "It is important that the relatives be contacted immediately," or "Get this patient out as soon as you can. We need the bed."

In some departments of a hospital, in some institutions, emphasis is placed upon obtaining a careful social history, or "life history." This is especially true of psychiatric hospitals or services. Departments of pediatrics and rehabilitation in some health care facilities also require careful history and interviews with relatives. Somewhere in their training, most medical students are taught to take a "history," with emphasis upon significant medical problems. They are also told of the importance of obtaining a history of the patient's background and of interviewing close relatives, but more often than not the medical chart has such entries as the following: F.l.& w, M.d. (CVA) Sibs. l. & w. Occasionally the patient's employment is noted.

Social work students in graduate schools spend a great deal of time learning how to take a social history and how to utilize it in understanding and in helping a patient; but while they often go through the ritual of obtaining a social history, they frequently fail to take the second step; the use of it in understanding and helping their patient. The social history lies buried and often forgotten in a file drawer. Some schools of social work and psychology put the major emphasis upon the relationship with the patient and upon his present situation, rather than upon his past. *All are important, the past, the present, and the relationship, when one is trying to help and understand people.* And the family may be an important resource to use not only in understanding but in healing the patient.

However, as we have already observed, only at the time when something is needed, the moment of crisis, are relatives recognized. Usually they are ignored, avoided by the staff, often made to feel they are in the way. Ask any nursing home proprietor what is her biggest problem and almost always she will say, "the relatives." "Why?" "They interfere. They try to tell us how to care for the patients. 'My father won't eat fried foods.' 'My mother likes a cup of tea and toast in the afternoons.' As if we had time to provide special diets. . . ." They call at inconvenient times to ask, "How is my father doing? Do you think he is going to get any better?" Another administrator said, "Sometimes the families will take out a patient, let him eat foods not on his diet and sometimes get him drunk. Then they bring him back to the nursing home and we are supposed to care for him while he sobers up."

Why do families do these things? "Guilt, I suppose." "What does that mean?" The administrator shrugs her shoulders. "What can be done with the families?" "We don't have enough time or staff to take care of patients, let alone their families. We do the best we can."

abandonment or desertion

Another nursing home administrator said:

Not only do families get in the way, but I find the reverse is also true. They are never there when they are needed. A patient runs out of medicine and it may take two or three days to locate the relative and get the prescription filled. One of the biggest problems is the problem of abandonment or desertion of the patient. Most of our patients are elderly and many no longer have any close relatives. If they are well enough to be aware of what is going on, it is very hard on them when other patients have visitors and they never do. We try to get volunteers in to visit with these patients but while this helps they never take the place of the family. I remember one case, a woman dying of a

*brain tumor. The hospital had referred her and sent her
father over to make the arrangements for her admission.
He was a tall, very erect old man who introduced himself
as Colonel Edward (not his real name). He was cold and
businesslike. He wanted a private room for his daughter
and made no objections to the charges. Once they were
completed he asked to see the room, but did not go
inside—just stood in the doorway and looked around. He
didn't say a word but turned and walked down the hall
and gave a brief look into the dining room and the lounge.
"I will bring my daughter over tomorrow," he said not
looking at me as he started toward the lobby. He had spent
less than twenty minutes in the place. Usually families
want to see everything, feel the mattress on the bed, check
out the bathroom, go through the dining room, and even
the kitchen. They want to know who takes care of the
patients at night, how often the doctor comes, and who
will call them if the patient gets worse. You get used to
families wanting to know these things, and it surprises
you when one of them doesn't.*

*The Colonel brought his daughter in the next day, in-
troduced her to me and said to her, "This is a well-run
place, very clean. You will like it here." Then he wheeled
around and marched out of the room. I was left to tell the
daughter that this was a nursing home and her father
had made arrangements for her to stay here. She took it
very well. "It would have been better if father could have
told me himself," she said quietly, "but he's so proud and
this is very hard on him."*

*She never mentioned him again, poor thing. A check came
promptly the first of every month, but the Colonel never
once visited his daughter. When visitors came to see the
other patients, I would see her look at them hungrily, and
then turn her head away and close her eyes. I called him
two or three times to ask him to come and see her. "Does
she need anything?" he would ask. "She needs to see you,"*

*I would reply, and I admit I spoke sharply. "Thank you,"
he would say stiffly and hang up. This patient deteriorated
very rapidly and lived only a few months. When she died
her father sent the undertaker to claim her body and I
understand he gave her a wonderful funeral. Families!
Don't talk to me of families. The things I could tell you
about some of them!*

There is no way of knowing how this proud old man really
felt about his daughter and her illness. No one knew what they
had meant to each other before she became ill. Was he, in
spite of his apparent coldness, so deeply attached to her that
he was unable to bear her suffering, or had they reached an
understanding in their relationship—this daughter and
father—so that this was not a desertion but an arrangement
they both accepted and understood? Did the physician, the
nurse, social worker, or anyone give these two an opportunity
to talk of their feelings about this illness and plan with them, or
if such an offer was made, was it refused by the father and also
the daughter? No one will ever know. All that is known is that a
woman was brought to a nursing home by her father. He paid
for her care but never returned to see her and she died alone.
On the basis of these meager facts a judgment was made that
she was abandoned.

legal and ethical problems

Such cases as this are a severe test of the health worker's ability
to remain nonjudgmental, and there are many of them. Any big
city hospital can cite numerous cases. One was an old man,
unconscious, brought into the emergency room by a man and
woman who claimed to be his daughter and son-in-law. They
gave information as to his name, address, and social security
number, and then before the doctor had examined the old
man, they disappeared. Investigation proved that the address
was fictitious. The social security number was inaccurate. The
man and woman were never located. The old man did not
regain consciousness and the hospital had legal problems to

untangle—who would be responsible for authorizing any necessary surgery, and when he died, as he did shortly after admission, who was to take responsibility for burying him?

In a Midwestern hospital a patient was referred in by a physician in a remote county for evaluation and diagnosis. When these were completed a nursing home was recommended, but the relatives refused to sign the appropriate papers. "He is too sick for a nursing home. He should stay in the hospital," they said and in spite of all the efforts of the members of the staff—the social worker, the physician, the hospital administrator—the family refused to relent. Here again, the hospital was faced with both legal and ethical problems. The patient was too ill to be discharged. None of the staff had the authority to place him in a nursing home when there were legally responsible relatives who could authorize this. The relatives had not abandoned the patient. They were quite solicitous and visited him frequently. The hospital and the family were deadlocked. "If this gets out," the hospital administrator said distractedly, "We could have the whole hospital full of chronically ill patients." "It's just another example," one of the doctors growled, "of families deciding what kind of treatment the patient needs." "If you had referred the family to us at the time of admission," the social worker said in a superior tone of voice, "we might have been more helpful. It is never good to refer families at a time of crisis." "Very well," said the administrator. "Hereafter we'll automatically refer *all* families to your department." "Not unless you give me money for more staff," retorted the social worker and thus internal problems as well as external ones were reactivated, while the innocent cause of all this ill-natured hassling was mercifully too ill to be aware of it.

The relatives of other patients for whom admission was sought found in the next few weeks they were subjected to an unusually rigorous interrogation. They were questioned as to their willingness to accept and take responsibility for carrying out whatever recommendations were made by the hospital.

Families were understandably irritated and relations between them and the hospital were not improved by this incident. "You would think that at the very least we were irresponsible, scheming, conniving creatures who planned only to dump our mother and take off," one woman said bitterly. "We wouldn't have made the effort to bring her here if we hadn't cared for her."

reasons for desertion and abandonment

Abandonment or desertion remains a serious problem especially where the patient is chronically ill or handicapped and requires some form of custodial care. Nursing homes and mental hospitals have the largest number of such patients. A social worker in one of the large state hospitals discussed this.

There are many reasons for this. When the patient is first admitted, most relatives visit once a month or oftener, but as time passes and he shows little improvement and all indications are that he will not recover, the visits become less frequent and eventually cease. Now, mind you, I am speaking of the chronically ill patient. Abandonment is not as great a problem with the acutely ill. There are exceptions, of course, among the families of the chronically ill. Frequent visits are difficult for most families. Like many of the older hospitals, this one is in an isolated area, reached only by car or bus. For some families the trip is a financial hardship. In other cases illness may occur, the closest relatives may die, and the younger members of the family feel little responsibility for visiting someone they scarcely knew. Sometimes a family moves out of the state. The reasons for failing to keep contact with the patient may be quite logical, but we are left with a patient who, as far as we are able to judge, is abandoned. And these people do not do well. Even the ones who seem unaware of their surroundings sense that something is wrong. They are more likely to be restless and irritable, or they may withdraw into some inner world of their own and respond to no one. The ones who do know what is happening get very anxious and upset. Even though they may understand the reasons why they have no visitors they keep hoping someone will come. Some of the letters they write are heartbreaking. Sometimes they will make up stories which they tell to us or the other patients to explain why no one visits. "My wife has a very important position and she can't get away just now," one old man used to explain. Actually his wife was dead and although he had been told this he could not accept it. Another patient explains, "My daughter is away on a little visit. She will come and see me just as soon as she gets back." This 'little visit' has lasted six years. The daughter moved out of the state. She sometimes writes and sends money but she has not been back to visit. Still another patient is very jealous of her companions who have visitors and is sometimes abusive and disruptive. "Why do you want anyone to come and see you in a place like this? Your people only come so they can laugh at you and make fun of you. I won't allow anyone to visit me." And then likely as not she bursts into tears.

Asked if the staff had regular or sustained contacts with the relatives she shook her head.

No. After the initial interview the professional staff see very little of the relatives. If there is some problem relating to the patient's care, we do of course, try to locate them. None of us refuses to see the relatives, but we leave it up to them to take the initiative.

Relatives are acutely aware of this situation. As one puts it:

I ask to see the doctor and I usually can if I wait long enough, although sometimes it means I miss the 4 o'clock bus. When I do get in to see him he doesn't exactly tap the desk with his pencil but he seems to have a lot on his mind. He answers my questions but he is kind of vague. He never asks me what I think of my husband, if I have noticed any changes. If I say "He doesn't seem as confused today," he answers, "He will have good and bad days, but don't expect much change in him." I try to find out if I can do anything for him, if I can take him home for the weekend. "We will see. A little later perhaps. Keep coming to visit him." I don't expect a miracle. I gave up on that a long time ago. But my husband and I were married for thirty-five years and we were very close. I'd like to feel now that there was something I could do that meant something. He is still my husband. But I feel that the staff doesn't know or care whether I visit or not. They act as if I have nothing to contribute. Maybe I'm exaggerating my importance, but that's the way I feel.

what would help families

The daughter of a college professor spoke of this problem one day. Her father had been in a nursing home and was now in a mental hospital.

I do not believe that the staff of nursing homes or mental hospitals have any understanding of how families feel, but I suppose that statement is not really fair. Some of them must have awareness of what relatives go through, but they certainly conceal it. We are made to feel that their only interest in us is the money we can provide. Other than that, we are in the way, to be avoided if possible. I can understand why patients are "abandoned" by their families. I know what a physical effort it is to make myself visit my father whom I loved very much. I think every time I go how futile it is. Most of the time he doesn't even know me. When I look at him, a frail old man who can take only a few trembling steps, who cries easily although I don't know whether it is from sorrow or not, I think this isn't the father I once knew. I think he died when he had his second stroke.

It's the memories, you see, that tear me apart. Whenever I see him I can't keep from remembering what he once was.

In all fairness, the nursing home staff or the people at the hospital where he is now never knew him when he was well. And I suppose they see so many like him that they forget that these poor souls weren't always this way.

I think that there are two things that would help families: one, to be helped to feel they had some part in the care and the treatment of their relative other than just the writing of a check. Two, if there were someone they could talk to about their concerns, the way they felt about their relative and what has happened to him. Who would let you cry sometimes, and know you weren't just feeling sorry for yourself but that you just felt dreadfully alone and were just tired of trying to cope. I'm more fortunate than many of the families. I have a husband and a family. But I can't talk to my husband. He and my father were never very close and I feel he resents my visits to the hospital. The children, well, you know how children are—they have their own interests and they should. My brother is no help either. He has never visited my father. "My God, Ethel," he'll say, "I can't. I just can't." I can understand this, but it makes me angry and it frightens me, too, because if something happened to me there would be no one to come to see my father.

There was never anyone I could talk to after my father became ill—not in the first hospital when he had his first stroke, nor in the nursing home or the present hospital. There was a nurse once, an L.P.N. she called herself, in the nursing home. I talked to her a few times. She was terribly busy, but she listened. She was gruff, but kind, and she had a lot of common sense. I think she knew how I felt, but then my father got worse and was sent to this last hospital. In this place there is no one, or at least I haven't met anyone who seems to have the time or the interest. On the ward there is an attendant, a pleasant, friendly, little woman. She knows my father better than anyone else, and she will tell me little things about what he has been doing during the week. This helps and I am glad my father has her to look after him, but it's not exactly what I am looking for . . . for myself. I know I sound as if I were the patient, and sometimes I wonder . . ."

The mental hospital social worker was asked if she thought that more sustained contacts with the relatives would make abandonment of the patient less of a problem. She considered this. "Yes, I think it would help in some cases but," and she shook her head. "Do you find that some of the relatives need some kind of counseling?" "Oh yes," she said quickly. "We find some of the family members are sick or sicker than the patient. We try to refer them for counseling to an agency near their homes. I often wish," she said wistfully, "that we had as much staff as some of the outpatient clinics or psychiatry departments so we could provide the support they need. It would not only help them but the patients.

families' need for understanding

Even with staff available for more individual attention the relatives sometimes still feel frustrated, as does the staff. The reasons for this are varied. Sometimes, as in the following narrative, it seems to have been faulty communication. This is an excerpt taken from the diary of a woman whose husband had recently been admitted to the psychiatric ward of a general hospital as an acutely ill patient.

My husband, whom I have loved and who has loved me, is a stranger now and I know no way to reach him. I feel I am in some way responsible for his illness and yet I don't know how. I need someone to help me. I am afraid I'll say or do the wrong thing, but then my husband seems so far away. Sometimes I think nothing I can say or do will matter.

I have tried to talk to the doctor but he is brusque and noncommittal. He acts as if I am intruding in some way. I know he is supposed to be very good and I can only hope he gives my poor husband some of the warmth and under-standing he denies me. He keeps referring me back to the

*social worker—she is a young thing, very pretty, but I get
nothing from her which helps. She takes a social history
which she explains is to help in understanding my husband. I try very hard to answer all her questions although
I am not accustomed to speaking of such intimate matters.
I watch her write down my answers in her neat handwrit-
ing. She is as precise and exact in this as in her questions,
but, I think, how can words with their many meanings
really describe a relationship between two people? I try to
say this to her but she just looks at me flatly and says, "We
find it is helpful to talk about one's problems." I ask about
my husband's condition, "What should I expect, what
should I do?" "It is hard to tell. We have not completed all
our tests. Oh yes, you can visit. We encourage the families
to keep in touch with the patients."*

*I am wondering if this is the kind of therapy the staff feels
is best for the families, or if the social worker just doesn't
know. I feel as if I am stumbling through this experience
with no one to help me. My husband is the most important.
He needs all the help he can get if he is to get well, but
what can I do, what should I do?*

Asked if she recalled this woman, the young social worker
thought a moment. "Oh yes," she said, "she was very upset
but I was never able to establish a relationship with her."

As much as she needed help, was this woman too
distraught to be able to use it or to understand it was being
offered, or was the social worker not sensitive enough or
skillful enough to communciate her concern and understanding? Communication between two people flows both ways and
often is an uneven and uncertain process.

interference

Interference was another term used by the nursing home
administrator to describe the problems with families. It covers
many kinds of situations. There is the one where so many

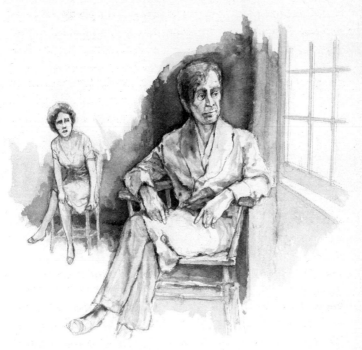

FIGURE 6
> "My husband, whom I have loved and who has loved me, is a
> stranger now and I know no way to reach him."

relatives crowd into the patient's hospital room that, as one
nurse said tartly, "you have to crawl over them to empty the
patient's bedpan." "Oh yes," she added, "we have visiting
hours but some families pay these no mind. I don't want the
nurses turned into a police force, but sometimes things get
tense around here."

Sometimes families think they are doing no harm but in
actuality are undermining a treatment plan. An example of this
are the relatives who bring in food to a patient on a special
diet. This frequently happens and sometimes can create complications if the patient, for instance, should be scheduled for a

series of gall-bladder studies. An instance where the parents thought they were doing the right thing is illustrated by the following incident.

how one family was helped

On the rehabilitation service a teen-ager was admitted who had severe back and leg injuries as a result of an automobile accident. It was felt that with proper treatment there was a good chance he would recover. Orders were written for daily treatment by the physical therapist. He was to be up in a wheelchair for much of the day and encouraged to do as much as possible in self-care. One or the other of the parents, however, was almost constantly at the boy's bedside or seated next to his wheelchair. They tried to anticipate his every need. "Oh, don't move, I'll get that! Be careful," they would say.

The chief physiatrist, observing the parents on rounds one morning, was mildly profane. "Damn it! If this isn't stopped, this kid will never walk. Has anyone spoken to the parents?"

The nurse said, "We were waiting for you to do that, doctor."

He gave her a long, level look. "Hmm!" he muttered, then he added, "But all of you have to help with this. You," he said to the physical therapist, "show the father how to give the exercises. And you," he said to the nurse, "give these parents a little love. They are scared." To the attendant he said, "Encourage the mother to let the boy wheel himself. Keep an eye on him. If he gets too tired, take over. Yes, I'll talk with the parents first," he concluded. Starting off, he turned back to say, "We'll talk about families in the Tuesday seminar." The mother of the boy spoke of the doctor's talk with them.

"We thought we were doing the right thing, but I guess we had been so scared, we weren't using good sense. After all, he is our only child. I knew the staff didn't like our being

here so much, but we couldn't stay away, we simply couldn't.

"The doctor understood this but he put things in a different kind of focus. He made us feel we were needed. He showed us some of the things we could be doing, and he drew a picture showing us where the injuries were and then he explained about the treatment. Now we know what we can do. We'll make mistakes because we'll still get scared, but there is hope now. We have to learn all over again what every parent has to learn—to let go but be there when we are needed."

neglect or mistreatment

Families and the health workers face many problems in the process of learning how to work together. Too hasty a judgment as to the motivations of either group may not only be unfair, but may lead to further misunderstanding. Confronted with the illness of a member of their family, relatives can quickly lose their objectivity, and the health workers, deeply involved in caring for many sick people, can also lose their perspective. For example, it takes rigid self-discipline on the part of the health worker not to react with anger when he encounters situations where there appears to have been neglect or mistreatment of patients by their relatives. Nowhere in the hospital are there more examples of this than on a pediatric ward. A child is brought in severely malnourished and the staff's first reaction is, "Why did the family let the child get in this condition?" rather than feeling pity and sadness for a family where there is great deprivation and poverty. Another child is brought in who has been bitten several times by a rat, and again the initial reaction is often, "Where was the mother, why wasn't someone around to protect this child?" Only someone who has lived in a ghetto can understand how difficult it is to maintain a twenty-four-hour vigil against such attacks.

The "abused child" brings forth an especially strong

reaction by the staff, professional and nonprofessional. This term is used to describe the children brought into a hospital with severe injuries where there is only a vague or unsatisfactory explanation as to how they acquired them. "He fell off the bed," or "I was asleep and don't know what happened." Often examination of these children reveals old fractures, never treated, and numerous scars which appear to have been from beatings. All are indications of severe neglect or mistreatment. Investigation usually reveals that the parents are responsible. In some instances the parents are young and ignorant, or they may have lived such desperate lives themselves that they are only treating the child as they, themselves, were treated. In some instances, one or both of the parents are found to be mentally ill, perhaps dangerously so.

In all these examples, the parents are extremely sensitive to the staff's reactions and if they feel there is any anger or criticism of them, they may not allow the baby to remain in the hospital as long as necessary or may fail to keep subsequent clinic appointments. They may become surly and hostile and resent any recommendations the staff makes if they feel they are being blamed for the baby's condition. Even though the staff's suspicions are correct in the case of the "abused child"—that the parents are responsible—it is extremely important that the staff, every one of them, maintain a nonjudgmental attitude. The parents of these children are wary and suspicious. They have usually had negative previous experiences with social agencies or legal authorities. If any member of the staff allows his anger to spill out, the parents may take the baby and disappear before legal protection for the infant can be arranged. Sometimes they surface at another hospital months later, and the baby has new injuries or may be dying. Usually in such cases as these, it takes skilled counseling to get such parents to accept help for themselves and for them to permit proper treatment for the child.

other problems presented by families

Families present many other kinds of problems. The "overprotective mother" needs little discussion. The reasons for her behavior are many and complicated. Ideally she should be referred to a skilled therapist, but if she can be aided even in very small ways to "let go" and permit her child more freedom, he and she both will benefit. Here the health worker may be able to help. "Let's see if your little boy can feed himself. It's all right if he gets food all over everything. We are used to that," or "I'll look in on him and be sure he's asleep before I go off duty," or "I'll stay with him for a little while after you leave."

Some relatives frankly would like to see the patient dead and buried and make little effort to conceal their feelings. Knowing nothing of what has created such an attitude, the health worker needs to proceed cautiously. Maybe the patient justly deserves this reaction, but the health worker cannot judge this. To him, this is a patient who needs a certain kind of care and his responsibility is to provide it.

There are also the relatives who are "sicker than the patient." They are often the relatives of the psychiatric patient, but not exclusively so. They may be related to the patients on any service. Sometimes, in the best interest of the patient, they may have to be barred from the patient's room. This kind of decision must be made by someone in authority but the health worker's observations of the interaction between the patient and his relatives may aid the professional staff in identifying such a problem. "This patient always seems so upset after his family visits him," or "I don't know why it is, but the patient seems afraid of his father. He said he didn't want to see him anymore."

utilization of families

Most families, even ones with serious problems, can be utilized in the care of the patient. It is well to remember that whether they are a good or bad influence upon the patient they were a part of his life before he became ill and will be when he is discharged. To treat a patient as if he came from nowhere, and would vanish into the unknown if he recovered, is not good medicine no matter where it is practiced. It would be good if it could be said that utilization of the family into the treatment plan for the patient was integrated into the very bones and muscles of medical practice. Many physicians do practice this, but equally as many do not. Administrators, overwhelmed by too many patients and too little staff, see only the negatives of family involvement.

health worker's role

If the health worker is in a health care setting where this concept of involving the family in the care and treatment of the patient is practiced, he is indeed fortunate, and will have little difficulty in knowing what he should do. However, if he is not in such a setting, he may have to be the instigator of family involvement. As he observes the family when they visit the patient, he should be able to make some assessment of the positives and negatives of the relationship which exists between them. Some of his observations may alert the rest of the staff and enable them to provide better care for the patient and his family. Or he, the health worker, may utilize his observations to modify his own behavior with the relatives. Instead of resenting their presence, and showing this by impatience or rudeness, he may pick up positives he has observed. For example, he may say "Your father was so pleased with the birthday card you sent him. He showed it to everyone." Or he may help the families feel more comfortable with the patient and give them a sense of being useful and needed by such comments as, "Your father would be pleased if you asked him to show you what he has done in the woodworking shop this last week," or "Your mother is always more relaxed and easier to care for after you visit." Little things, as has been noted before, cement or destroy good relationships.

Sometimes a search for positives in the relationship between a patient and his family may seem to be a fruitless task. All the ingenuity and imagination of the health worker may be severely taxed. There will be some cases where there is only hatred and self-interest. But it is well to remember that many people, because of their personality, their upbringing, and their cultural background, cannot show their tender feelings. It is possible the Colonel who never visited his daughter in the nursing home was one of these. Some Scandanavians are described as people of "fire and ice"; ice on the outside but full of the deepest emotions which they seldom show. There are often unknown threads of communication, of question and answer, of love given and received between a family and one of its members which may not be identified by the casual observer. The importance of being nonjudgmental cannot be stressed too strongly.

SUMMARY: The "moment of crisis" is never the ideal time to establish rapport with the patient's family. It may be unavoidable, if the patient's needs are urgent and imperative, but it is far better if the health care staff and the relatives are in good communication before an emergency arises. Any administrator of a health care facility, whatever its nature, will say that *care of the patient is the first priority,* and no one will quarrel with this objective, but *a good working relationship with relatives* is a part of this priority. Since the health worker is involved in so many aspects of patient care, he is in a unique position not only to identify potential problems between relatives and the patient but also to aid in their resolution. Should he ever experience great frustrations, let him remember that relatives, too, are often baffled and annoyed by the behavior of the health care staff.

ASSIGNMENT: Review your impressions and knowledge of the families of your last five patients. Make an assessment of the positive and negative aspects of the relationship between the relatives and the patient in all these cases, and decide what you can do in each of them to help the family and the patient.

3 the health worker and health care

"They're just people, Ma'am. . . ."

"Sometimes it's the only job. . . ."

"My son, the doctor."

"My mother is a nurse."

". . . it's just a feeling. . . ."

"I just *love* working with sick people. . . ."

"It's so easy to fool yourself."

8 who are the health workers?

The author looked up from the papers on her desk. "Since we are writing this book for health workers, I wonder if we shouldn't know more about them, who they are, where they come from, and how they happened to enter the health field."

"They're just people, Ma'am, no different from anyone else," the health worker said boredly.

"Perhaps, but I still wonder. . . ."

diversity of health care system

Someone once compared the health care system to an over-sized patchwork quilt full of holes, the holes being the areas not covered by any kind of health services. Nonetheless, the health care system is so large, so varied, so complex that many different kinds of people can be utilized, from the least skilled to the most highly specialized of scientists. This diversity of health workers is the first thing which impresses the observer: the difference in background, the dissimilarity in education, and the variety of experience. "You name it, we have it," a personnel director said, "from grandmothers to high school dropouts."

"Yes," the author said, "I agree there is diversity in the people in the health field and this variety is one of the strengths of health care programs and is at the same time

a challenge to the staff responsible for training. To create out of a large, unwieldy, totally dissimilar group of people a work force which provides care for the sick and the injured is quite an achievement. However, I think I am more interested in looking at the people themselves and why they choose health care as a career."

"Sometimes it is the only job," the health worker said grimly.

"Sometimes, perhaps during periods of high unemployment, but not always. . . ."

It must be understood, however, that the purpose for discussing the motivations which lead one into health care is *that they may affect the health worker's relationship and interaction with patients, their families, and other staff members.* An example of this is the laboratory technician who was refused admission to the school of nursing. She does not function well. She is resentful and angry. She feels as if her position is inferior to her original goal. She is so preoccupied with her own feelings, she is insensitive or unaware of the needs of patients or other staff members.

Now to look at some of the most frequently expressed reasons for entering the health field. If the health worker examines these carefully, he may see reflections of himself or, through them, he may be able to reevaluate his own motivations and measure them against the needs of the patients.

family pressure

An example of family pressure is that of a pharmacology clerk. His father, a storekeeper, after a lifetime of humiliations and frustrations, longed to be able to say with a pathetic kind of pride, "My son, the doctor." The story told by the son follows:

My father didn't realize it, but the pressure was terrific. He'd say, "Of course, the boy is free to choose, but. . . ." As I grew up I didn't protest too much. I received a certain amount of respectful attention from the relatives—as someone set apart, like the kid who is going to be a priest—and I unashamedly capitalized on this. I used to daydream a lot about being a doctor—saving lives and making ponderous pronouncements about matters of life and death. When I got in college, though, I found I didn't do well in most of the premed courses. I didn't like them. In fact, some of them, like the one where I dissected frogs, turned my stomach. But now, chemistry, I really dug that. So I end up as a pharmacy clerk and I like it. It's kind of a compromise with my father's wishes. I wear a white coat which pleases him and he can say I work in one of the biggest hospitals in the city. I suspect he leaves the impression I am running the joint.

Sure, he was disappointed, but it's my life and I couldn't see spending a lot of years doing something I didn't like. I've known fellows who did that and I feel sorry for them. My father's now working on my boy. "Maybe my grandson will be a doctor," he says. The kid's a nice guy, but kind of dumb. I'm afraid the old man's in for another disappointment. Too bad he couldn't have been a doctor himself.

Family pressure to choose a vocation is difficult to withstand, particularly so where the family means well and where there is a good relationship between parent and child. In this instance, the son was able to withstand his father's wishes and make his own decision. This may have been a compromise but, if so, the son seems to have made a good adjustment.

Sometimes the family's and the child's wishes coincide and both are happy. In other instances, the son or daughter who yields to the family's desires finds that in spite of himself, he comes to like his work. However, in a people-oriented field such as health, where good interrelationships with people are so important, the choice of vocation should never be a haphazard process. If possible, the decision should be made only after carefully considering the positive and negative aspects of the work. "Vocational misfits" do not usually make good employees.

someone they most admire

Often the first awareness of health care as a career comes from association with someone who is already working in the field. "My mother is a nurse." "My best friend is a lab technician." "Our family doctor was the greatest. I knew I wasn't smart enough to study medicine, but I thought there were things I could do for sick people." If these associations provide an opportunity for the health worker to learn something of both positives and negatives, he is in a good position to decide whether he wishes to choose health care as a career. Sometimes though, these are the people who tend to glamorize the field or to see only the superficial aspects such as the uniforms, the drama, the status symbols. Careful evaluation of motivation is important. "We try to help every applicant look carefully at his reasons for choosing health care as a career," the personnel director said somewhat defensively, "but you must remember that we are often under great pressure to fill positions. Sometimes," she concluded gloomily, "we are just grateful if a 'warm body' comes through our doors."

personal experience with illness

Many people enter the health field because they or some member of their family has had some experience with illness or injury. Because of their knowledge of the feelings and problems of patients, they can often make important contributions to health care. However, much depends upon how they adjusted to the illness of themselves or a family member. The LPN whose husband had rheumatoid arthritis said she was irritated with him because she felt he did not help himself enough.[1] Had she felt the same irritation toward the patients she cared for, this attitude could have been serious.

In another instance, a young girl, a former polio victim, had spent several years in a hospital and had come to feel more

[1]See the section on the only job (p. 157).

deeply attached to it than to her own home. She had several close and very satisfying relationships with various members of the staff. These had been very important and necessary while she was adjusting to a quite severe handicap. When she decided to apply for work in the hospital and expressed a wish to be assigned to the same ward on which she had been a patient, the question arose whether she was attempting to prolong her dependence upon the health care system. Perhaps not. It may have been only a very natural and human desire to be near the staff she was so indebted to, but it was important to know whether she had made the transition from "receiving to giving."

If she is truly to help the patients she cares for, the health worker must always be able to give more than she receives. This is difficult. Sometimes the health worker may be unaware that her own needs predominate and even if she is aware the appropriate adjustment is never easy. Sometimes counseling with someone who is an expert in health care is helpful.

difficulty in describing attraction of health care field

A young physical therapist says:

It's hard to put into words the reasons why you chose this kind of work and why you stay in it. Whatever you say sounds utterly stupid. All I know is that you go home after a day when everything has gone wrong and you swear you'll never go back, for anything or anybody. And you go over all the negatives. The bad-tempered resident who never remembers your name. The nurse who is always too busy to answer your questions. The treatment room that is always too crowded. The way patients are brought in without a single note in their charts to tell you what the doctor wants you to do and by the time you locate him it is almost closing time. Oh, you pile up quite a list.

But what happens? Something pulls you back. The pa-

tients? Well, they are a part of it. Even if what you do for them is not much somebody has to do it and you feel, well, you feel useful.

Another physical therapist overheard the above remarks and commented:

I think that's very low key. Maybe that's the way you want it, but I would put it like this. I've had days too when everything seemed to go wrong. The patients aren't cooperating. My own peer groups are not supporting. It seems as if the professionals, the doctors and the nurses, are not helping the patients. I feel as if everything is falling down on top of me. I go home ready to give up.

But when the next day comes, something really pulls you together. You get up and go to work. I don't know why. You just do. I don't know whether it's the patients or the thing inside of you. You can't let yourself down any more than you can let down the patients. Then too, you've had time since yesterday to look at things more objectively. You know that certain personal problems may have influenced your feelings. You think maybe the other members of the staff were having problems also. Maybe if you can discuss the difficulties with them, they can be worked out. Today, you feel, will be different. Things can't possibly be as bad today as they were yesterday.

I don't know if I've really said what I mean. It really is difficult to put something into words that have real meaning. Perhaps because we so seldom do. Suppose you just say it's just a feeling and leave it at that.

It is often true that the most sensitive people with the deepest feelings are the ones least able to express themselves. Others speak glibly of wanting to help people. They use the right words but what of the feeling?

As the personnel director says sharply:

How do you tell in one interview or in two or three what is real and what is phony? Take the young woman who comes in and says with a bright smile, "I just love working with sick people," and believe me I've had people say just that. What would you do with her! What do I do? Well, I am inclined to be pretty short with her. It's a stupid remark. But then I try to find out if she really is that shallow by asking about other experiences she has had and how she feels about them. Sometimes I try her out in a job where I think she won't do too much harm, a file clerk for example, but keep my fingers crossed. Sometimes such a person surprises me and turns out to be much more sensitive than I ever thought possible. You can't always tell. . . .

the only job

As the health worker said at the beginning of this chapter, sometimes entrance into the health field is out of necessity. The personnel director tells of one situation he knew about:

A middle-aged woman came into my office one day looking for work. She looked frail and appeared tired and discouraged. She told me that as a young woman she had worked briefly as a nurse's aide, then had married and quit when her first child was born. Now her children were grown. Only one was still at home. Her husband had rheumatoid arthritis and had been bedfast for several years. Finances were a problem because there was only a small pension and social security.

"I'm not trained to do anything, but I thought maybe I could do some kind of night work when my daughter can be home with my husband."

"Health care has changed a great deal," I told her. "You will have a lot to learn."

"I know," she said, "but I'm willing to try."

I had a lot of questions about whether she was strong enough and whether she could adjust to full-time work after all these years, but I put her on the rehabilitation ward temporarily.

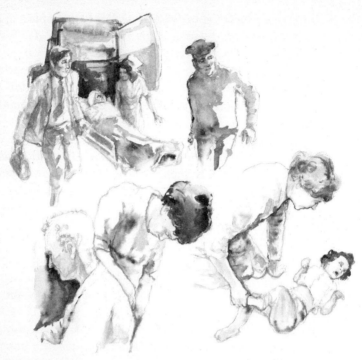

FIGURE 7
   One of the great strengths of the health field is the diversity of
   its staff.

*Five years later she is still there, but in the meantime she
has received on-the-job training and is now an LPN. She
told me later that the first few weeks were very difficult
and, more than once, she almost quit.*
*"But we needed the money—and you know, I found I was
really glad to get out of the house. My husband had gotten
on my nerves. I thought he complained too much and that
he didn't try hard enough to help himself. I can't say this
was ever an easy job, but I've learned a lot. I know how to*

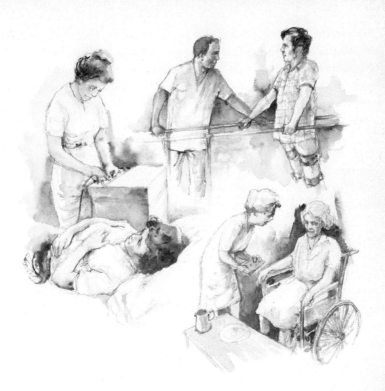

take better care of my husband—lots of little things I never
would have thought of which make him more comfortable.
And I have a better understanding of what he is going
through now that I have worked with other patients like
him. I know now that if I were in his place I would do a lot
more fussing than he ever has. You know, no one really
ever sat down and explained much about his illness—
what he was going through and what I could expect to
have happen. Even if they had, it wouldn't have meant as
much as it has to work in a place like this and see for
myself what happens to these patients and see how the
staff treats them. . . ."

Examples why health care was chosen for a career could
be continued, but these should be sufficient to stimulate

introspection on the part of the health worker. "How do you
know what your reasons are?" one queried. "It's so easy to
fool yourself." This is true but the health worker should make
an honest effort to discover them; first, because as has already
been noted, they may profoundly affect his interpersonal
relationships in the health field and secondly, the wrong
choice of a career, whatever it is, may be both a damaging and
a self-destructive experience for him. Motivations can be
complex and often contradictory. Sometimes one chooses a
health career for a poor reason and yet finds a satisfying and
productive place for himself. The LPN whose motivation was
one of necessity—not necessarily a poor one—found a good
life for herself. A good motivation such as the desire to learn
may turn out badly if, in pursuing this objective, the rights of
others are disregarded. An example of this is the medical
student in Chapter 5, the section on right to withhold information, who was oblivious to the needs of his patient. The wish to
help sounds like a worthy objective, but if it is primarily for the
purpose of enhancing one's self-image, it can be valueless and
sometimes harmful.

SUMMARY: One of the great strengths of the health field is
the diversity of its staff—diversity in terms of race or culture,
education, and geographical background. This diversity plus
the great variety in kinds of work requiring unskilled and
highly specialized people can create problems, human problems, when an effort is made to meld them into a pliable and
productive group of employees.

   The motivations leading people into health care are only
one aspect of this problem, but a highly important one
affecting all areas of interpersonal relationships. Determining
the true motivation or motivations is in itself a difficult task and
while the responsibility for this determination rests in large
part upon the shoulders of the health worker, he should not be
discouraged if he at first fails to identify the real reason he
chose the health field.

ASSIGNMENT: This assignment is a little different from the others you have done. Take these questions and see how many you can answer.

1 Why are you in the health field?
2 What do you think is your greatest asset in caring for patients?
3 What do you think is your greatest weakness in caring for patients?
4 What are some instances where your own interests got in the way of patient care?
5 Are you in the position you plan to stay in?

". . . the good old caste system. . . ."

"If I ran my business like this place is run. . . ."

"You don't want to look too dumb."

". . . it's the health workers who are right in there where the action is. . . ."

". . . it's the system that messes everything up."

". . . a 'facilitator.'"

"Doctors—they're really weird sometimes."

". . . 'a kindly old family doctor. . . .'"

". . . our survival technique."

". . . to walk alone. . . ."

9 the health worker and the health care system

The author and the health worker were having coffee together in the hospital cafeteria. The author looked around the room. "We have been talking about the great diversity of people in health care," she said thoughtfully. "The people in this room represent a good cross section of the field, at least in this kind of institution. We have students of all kinds, we have professionals, we have health workers, and we have patients."

The health worker in turn looked around and then returned to his coffee and doughnut. "Yeah," he said indifferently, "and the good old caste system is in full swing."

"Well look," he continued replying to the author's lifted eyebrow, "the doctors sit at one table by themselves. The medical students sit at another table by themselves. The nurses are by themselves. The technicians who wouldn't be caught dead associating with such people as the housekeeping staff are over in one corner. And the patients—do you see any of them sitting with any of the hospital staff?"

"Does this bother you?"

He shrugged. "It's just a fact of life, I guess," he replied matter-of-factly. "But when the administration comes out in the house bulletin and says we are just one big happy family, I have to smile."

The author looked troubled. "I am not trying to defend this system but I wonder if one of the reasons for it is that health care has grown so rapidly. There are so many different kinds of programs that even experts find it hard to keep up with all of them. Yet I am old enough to remember—you aren't—when most of the health care was provided by the family doctor. There weren't many nurses, there were no technicians, few laboratories, little research, none of all the elaborate and expensive equipment that health care facilities now take as a matter of course. I would like to think that as health care programs become more evenly distributed, some of these more objectionable features will disappear. Health care is still uneven and spotty. There are many places where the family doctor is still the major source for care and many patients in this country must travel a long distance in order to get modern up-to-date medical treatment." The author stopped, embarrassed. *"I had no intention of lecturing you, but I would like to add just one more thing. Granted that health care organizations still lack adequate social mobility, there is upward movement. Some doctors and nurses started out as attendants and nurses' aides. Look at some of our best people in research. Many of them began as technicians. Look at how many health workers are taking some kind of training so that they can move up into a better job or improve their skills in their present assignment. Look at yourself."*

The health worker grinned at her. *"You made your point, but I would still say it isn't the best way to take care of sick people."*

the best way

What is the best way to care for sick people? Experts cannot agree. Is it the training of more physicians, more personnel at all levels? Is it to develop more paraprofessional programs? Is it more clinics, more hospitals, more nursing homes, more group practice? Experts do agree that health care is uneven in quality. One public health physician said, "Patient care in this country has never been noted for its excellence except in an irregular and rather spotty fashion. With the advent of modern technological advances the evenness of health care has deteriorated rather than improved."

And what of the health care system, the administrative structure around which health care programs are developed? A system which its enemies and friends agree is complex, often inefficient, and frequently confusing. More then one angry patient has said as he fought his way through masses of red tape, trying to get an itemized statement of his bill, "If I ran my business like this place is run, I would be broke in a year's time." Within and without the system there are complaints. Physicians complain of too much paperwork. Staff often complain of poor working hours, contradictory orders. However, in spite of all the negatives of the health care system, and unquestionably there are many, it still manages to provide care for the sick. "Not always *good* care," says the public health physician, "but *fair*."

Discussion of the different ways of caring for the sick; the arguments for one method as against another; or a detailed study of the health care system, its origin, its development, its probable future, have a place in the training of the health worker. Knowledge of the methods and the functioning of the health care system will help the health worker keep his impressions of his own institution in appropriate balance. It may be that in order to get much information about these subjects he will have to take the initiative in searching out information from magazines, books, or special study groups.

focus of this chapter

In this chapter the emphasis will be, as it has been in the rest of the book, upon interpersonal relations. How the health worker learns about his own institution; how he develops ways of understanding and working with the staff, the professionals, the administration, and his coworkers. Finally, an effort will be made to determine how the health worker finds his own role in the health care system.

conventional ways

The newly employed health worker in the larger institutions will usually be given some form of orientation. He will view some films giving some information about the organization and kind of institution it is. These statements are usually quite general: "This is a 300-bed hospital for the treatment of the mentally ill." "This nursing home takes only ambulatory patients." Or, "This is a teaching hospital for the various disciplines of nursing, medicine, physical therapy, psychology. . . . Patients who are admitted are evaluated on the basis of whether they will be good teaching cases. Only referrals from a physician are accepted."

The health worker will also be given information about the names of the department heads. Staff benefits will be discussed: the working hours, the rate of pay for overtime, sick leave, insurance, what to do in case of an accident. Sometimes he will be given further briefing in the department to which he is assigned about his specific duties. Sometimes in this kind of instruction training manuals or audiovisual materials may be utilized. The health worker often comes away from these meetings vaguely dissatisfied and unable to put his dissatisfactions into words.

"I guess it's the best they can do," the health worker said resignedly, "but there are a lot of unanswered questions after one of those sessions. When you are new you don't like to ask too many questions. You don't want to look too dumb. I had worked in a couple of institutions, a nursing home and a mental hospital, before coming here, but I wasn't sure what they meant by teaching cases and I'll bet most of the people there didn't know. The training in the department went better, but I think they forgot that people

learn in different ways. Some workers like the training manuals, but I found them boring. Too much repetition. I got more out of asking my chief to explain the way that he wanted things done. He's a great guy, he doesn't mind answering questions, but all departments wouldn't have someone like him."

The health worker in the smaller institutions may not get any formal orientation. He will be fortunate if there is someone to explain his daily assignments, but he may be more fortunate than his counterpart in the larger facility because he often is a part of a closer knit group of employees with less formal structure, less rigid defining of assignments.

"I liked that part," the health worker said, "where everyone knew everyone else. If someone was sick, one of us would do his work. The director would talk over problems with us over coffee. Of course there wasn't much chance to advance there, and not any opportunity to learn, and the patients seemed pretty much alike. I wouldn't think that now, of course," he said quickly seeing the expression on the author's face, "but there is a lot more going on here, more of everything. . . ."

It would seem that in the smaller institutions it is easier to maintain good interpersonal relations between professional and nonprofessional staff, between staff and patients, and between the facility itself and the community. One administrator of a health department says that once an institution gets above a certain size it loses its ability to maintain close-knit or informal relationships among all its staff. Smaller groups develop and may compete with each other in large facilities. He cites as an example a hospital in a largely rural community. Most of the staff were from the same area although some of the physicians were from a neighboring city and were employed only part-time. As long as the hospital had only 150 beds, there was good morale and good communication. The administrator knew most of the employees by their first name. The atmosphere was a pleasant and friendly one and most of the patients spoke warmly of the care they received there. All this began to change when the hospital was enlarged to 250-bed capacity and a mental hygiene unit was added to it. The increased size meant a more formal administrative structure was necessary; some employees were brought in from other areas and some tensions and rivalries developed between the new and old staff. Patients and staff were not as happy, nor was the hospital administrator satisfied with the situation:

> *Yes, there are differences and I don't like some of them any more than the rest of the staff does. As we have expanded, we've had to set up a more rigid administrative structure and this means I don't have the personal contact with many of the staff which I used to have. I seem to find myself spending most of my time in some kind of meeting, budget hearings, planning conferences, board meetings. . . . I try to have regular staff meetings, but they aren't very productive. It ends up with my doing most of the talking. The staff doesn't even gripe much. A bad sign. I keep hoping when I get on top of all these changes and the whole operation settles down into a pattern that I can find some way of improving communication. Frankly I don't know how to do it now.*

The health worker read the above comments:

> *"I don't know that administrator, but I think he's lost his staff. They are never going to trust him again. I don't know what happened, but I can guess. I'll bet he forgot to take the staff along with him when he was making all those changes. He and the board probably got together and dreamed up this plan for making the hospital bigger, and then they went out and got the plan approved and found the money for it, but if he acted like most administrators, none of the staff, except for a few of the supervisors and department heads, were told one thing about the plan until it was all worked out. I don't care if the administrator and the board members have lived in that town all their lives, there's plenty the health workers could tell them*

about how patients feel, what they need. After all, it's the health workers who are right in there where the action is, all twenty four hours of it. Oh, well . . ." the health worker said, shrugging his shoulders, and he got up and walked out of the room.

The health worker had scored a point. While decision making, planning, and program development are tasks usually accomplished at a top administrative level, the health worker might have something of value to contribute to them. He sees health care from an entirely different point of view than the administrator or a board of trustees. He is closer to the patient and knows him better than anyone in the health care system. Does this suggest that better communication up and down the administrative chart might improve health care?

"I don't know whether it would improve health care," said the health worker coming back into the room, "but it would sure do a lot for the health workers."

it's the system

"How do you learn to get along with administrators?" the author asked.

"It isn't easy. If you have a good guy who likes people, you usually do all right. Usually, but not always. You see, it's the system that messes everything up. In the orientation lectures at this institution they hand out a sheet of paper called an organizational chart. Up at the top is the board of trustees. Under them is the administrator and under him are all the department heads. But believe me, that's not like it is.

"From where I sit, it looks like this. We have two bosses in this institution, the administrator and the doctors, and if the nurses get in the act, there are three: Let me show you what I mean:

"A doctor orders a neck brace for one of his patients. So one of the health workers takes the requisition slip down to the brace shop. The brace shop must have checked with the

administrator, because word comes back that the administrator says, 'Hold it. There's no money.' The doctor says, 'My patient needs that brace,' and he fires back another requisition. The brace shop says, 'No, not unless we get an OK from the administrator.' Then the nurse steps in. 'Let me handle this,' she says to the doctor. She goes and talks with the administrator and they must have worked out something, because the patient gets his brace. But it looks to me as if the doctor always wins."

"Where were you when all of this was going on?" the author asked.

"Me! I ducked out of sight. I wasn't going to get involved." The author sighed, "And the patient was somewhere in the middle of all that."

"So was the health worker."

"Was it actually a question of dual authority, or was this just poor communication?"

"Communication was part of it, I guess, but the way it looks to me is that the doctors run the hospital, but the administrator thinks he does, so they're bound to tangle sometimes."

The author looked doubtful. "I can see how it might look that way to you, but I suspect that there are better ways of describing the system. Let's see what the administrator says about it."

The administrator smiled when the health worker and the author told him why they wanted to see him.

"I can understand why you would be confused," he said to the health worker. "Most people are. My business associates can never understand how we manage to operate. We do, however, and strange as it may seem, the system works.

"You are correct," he told the health worker, "we do have a dual system of authority. Often this isn't shown on the administrative chart, which adds to the confusion. Every health care facility has what I would suspect," smiling at the health worker, "you would call a different mix of this combination of administrator and physician. The older pattern, and one still found in many places, is that a physician is the administrator. In many nursing homes a nurse is the administrator. One mental hygiene clinic I know is run by a psychologist. You will find, however, that in all these facilities, the care and treatment of patients is the physician's responsibility. Some parts of that care may be delegated by him to some other member of the professional team, such as a nurse, psychologist, social worker, physical therapist, or medical aide. However, none of the care and treatment of patients is ever the administrator's direct responsibility, for which I say 'Thank Heavens!'"[1]

"I see the administrator's role as that of a 'facilitator.' His job is to find the equipment and the personnel to handle all aspects of patient care, to create the environment in which the physician can practice. Physicians have never liked paperwork. If they had to do all the administrator does, they would have little time for their patients.

"Money to run health care institutions comes from many sources: fees, state and local governments, federal funds for research programs, trust funds, or programs such as medicare and medicaid. This money must be strictly accounted for. The administrator, with the help of his advisory group, must decide how it is to be budgeted."

The administrator stopped. "Here I am trying to describe the health care system in a few paragraphs, but let me just add that complicated as it is, it works because of the thing the author is always stressing—the interpersonal relationships. If there is understanding and appreciation of the separate roles of the administrator, the physicians, and the health care staff, the system can function. I think,

---

[1] A landmark decision in 1965, *Darling v. Charleston Community Hospital,* in Charleston, South Carolina, ruled that the hospital board of directors, and through them the administrator, was responsible for the quality of medical care provided patients.

however," he added, "our poorest communication is with the health workers."

"And patients," the author said quietly.

"Oh, yes. We have to find better ways of communicating with patients. There is so much we could learn from them." He turned back to the health worker, "Now, I have a question to ask you. Do you think that the health workers who are involved in patient care tend to side with the professionals if any differences arise with the administration?"

The health worker grinned, half embarrassed. "Guess we do."

"That would be natural. You work with them more closely. I find that I am more likely to be considered the 'bad guy' by your group. On the other hand, the health workers who are in such places as the admitting office or purchasing office are inclined to be on my side and see the professionals as the ones who always overspend, or make unreasonable requests. Well, all I ask is that you give me an even break.

"Before you go," he continued, "let me tell you about the neck brace. The brace shop was asked to hold the requisition until I could find out where the money was coming from. The doctor had failed to have that checked out before he sent in the requisition. If he had cleared it with his chairman, he would have found that the budget for that department was already overspent. It worked out all right, however. The social worker talked with the family and they were able and willing to pay for the prosthesis. If they hadn't been, the chairman and I would have gotten together and worked out something. You would be surprised at the miracles we sometimes produce."

Confusion about the functioning of the health care system is not uncommon. Some means should be developed within each facility to help the health worker understand the dual roles of the administrator and the physician. The latter's responsibilities are usually better understood although the health workers not directly associated with patient care may not have an accurate impression of them.

understanding doctors

"You've found it easier to understand doctors than administrators?" asked the author.

"Yes and no," the health worker replied. "They're pretty weird sometimes. You have to work at understanding them. When I first started as a health worker, I found I had to get rid of my image of a 'kindly old family doctor' who came to your home and gave you some pink pills out of his worn saddlebags and got you well. I never knew a kindly old family doctor. I think that was one of those fables handed down by my grandmother. We lived in the inner city when I was growing up. When we got sick, my mom packed us up and took us to the city hospital—a bus ticket and two transfers away. The clinics were always crowded and the doctors, well I don't remember any of them I would have described as kindly; efficient, yes, hurried, harassed, and overworked. Nor were any of them old. They were all young and thinking back now, I guess some of them were pretty scared of the patients who were older and more experienced than they were.

"In spite of experiences like this, I still clung to the old-family-doctor myth when I became a health worker and it took me a while to get over it. Then I found doctors were just people and I was mad at them for being human. There's still another thing. You ask around and you'll find a lot of health workers who once wanted to be a doctor. They didn't make it because they were too dumb, didn't have enough education or money, or something else happened. At any rate when we see some medical student

doing some stupid thing we think, 'If he made it into medical school, I could have too.' There's some feeling of resentment. From where we are it looks as if the doctors have everything—power, money, authority. But as we go along and have more experience, we see the hard work, the long hours, the kinds of responsibility—especially the responsibility—the doctors carry, and medicine begins to lose some of its glamour. That dream we had of being a doctor was just a dream. Most of us could never have followed through and made it into medical school.

"Anyway, once we get the image bit, the envy, and the daydreams out of the way, we get along pretty well with doctors. We do our thing. They do theirs."

The health worker has described some of his reactions to physicians but these do not fully describe what is often a complicated relationship between the physician and the rest of the health care staff. The physician, often because of his personality and surely because of his training, learns early to make decisions. He must have this ability. Indecisiveness where life and death issues are involved would be a disaster. Decision making, however, often involves other personnel in the health care system. Here the physician is less skillful. His training does not prepare him to translate his decisions into terms always understood by the health care staff, or more importantly engage their interest and cooperation. Unless he is an unusually perceptive and sensitive person, the physician learns how to develop good interrelationships only by trial and error. And in the process of learning, much resentment can be built up toward "his arrogant, authoritative ways." His commands of "Do this!" "Do that!" tolerate no failure. He, on the other hand, is filled with frustration, anger, and impatience with a staff too slow or indifferent to grasp what he sees so clearly. In such situations as the one just cited both physician and health worker may have need for a "troubleshooter," someone who can interpret the one to the other and help them both find a satisfactory solution for their problem. Often this role is the one assumed by or assigned to the nurse.

nurses and other professionals

Acting as the mediator is a function which the nurse had not anticipated when she chose her profession, nor did her training equip her to handle it. "It can be rough," one nurse said with a sigh, "not only do we act as a go-between for the health worker and physician, but we must also assume this role between the physician and his patient, between the administrator and the physician, and sometimes between the health care facility and the community. It takes all the psychology we have been taught and diplomacy which we have had to learn on the job. As is true of all middlemen, we can, and often do, end up pleasing no one."

"She does get it from both sides," the health worker agreed, "and if she sometimes lets us have it, I guess she has a right to. There was one nurse in the army. . . ." He grinned and then grew serious.

"I find it hard to keep up with what the nurses do. In one place, a mental hospital I worked in, they did mostly bedside nursing. In the nursing home I worked in, the nurse ran the place. Here in this hospital, I find them doing something different every day. It's confusing. . . ."

Nurses are the most innovative of the health care professionals. They have and are experimenting with new methods of patient care and they have also done a great deal of research—particularly in human relations. Probably the health workers directly involved in patient care feel closest to the nurses. The nurses often supervise them and also intercede when they get caught up in institutional red tape. Much of the inservice training for the health workers is provided by nurses.

The health worker usually has little to do with other professionals except on particular cases. But he needs to know something of the function of the various health professionals, such as the social worker and the psychologist.

the health worker's coworkers

"My coworkers? Oh, they are no trouble," said the health worker cheerfully. "Just as it is any place there are some people you like and some you don't like. We have our own small groups and we keep to those pretty much, not mixing with the others or the professionals. We have our own means of underground communication which we call our survival technique. It's our way of coping with the health care system. I guess that goes on everywhere."

Similar forms of communication do go on among all groups in the health care system and among the nurses and the doctors. Usually these groups, as the health worker indicated, have similar backgrounds and like interests. There is danger in this kind of informal communication, however, because misinformation and misinterpretations can be easily spread by this means. It is important in any facility that there be good channels of communication—official channels—which go up and down as well as across levels of operation.

patterns of conformity

In observing health workers as they go about their daily tasks one gets the impression that fairly quickly most of them settle into a round of routine procedures which vary little from day to day. "They develop a union mentality," one administrator said with some discouragement. "In their thinking and activity they rapidly become compartmentalized."

But what are the incentives for the health workers to break out of this pattern of conformity? There are few. In group meetings the health workers are encouraged to make suggestions as to ways of improving the institution's program but seldom do they speak up. One theory as to the cause of this problem is that the physicians have for so long been accepted as the "decision makers" in health care that the rest of the staff, professional as well as health worker, have first yielded and eventually lost their ability to make decisions. The hospital administrator feels that while this theory is one element in the problem of the staff's lack of initiative, the situation is far more complex:

Industry faces this same problem. Today you begin to hear reports of steps they are taking to involve more of their employees in the entire decision-making process. However, these programs are still largely experimental. In our health care institutions I think a big fault is in our training programs. We don't train employees to take initiative, to ask questions, to learn how to assume leadership roles. I think the administration has often been afraid to unlock such a door for fear things would get out of hand. One of the things that started me thinking about this was some of our group-sensitivity sessions. We have had quite a number of them for both our professional staff and our health workers. They have value. I think where they have been led by properly qualified people they have helped improve communication among staff and have created a sense of unity among individual groups. But the thing that I became aware of was that sometimes they seemed to destroy individual initiative. The individual members became too dependent on the group for the decision-making process. Some people say this is a basic problem of our entire educational system, that we do not help people to learn to "walk alone" and that when confronted with crisis situations many people cannot handle them appropriately. I am not sure of this but I would like in our inservice training programs to see some means developed to help our staff learn to do some independent thinking. I know, I am asking for trouble. But it would make my job much more interesting. And think how it might improve the whole health care system.

SUMMARY: It is ridiculous to think that one could cover the entire health care system, complicated and involved as it is, in one chapter. The topics selected for discussion seemed to be those in which the health worker might be most interested. While much of the discussion has been related to the larger institutions, the same problems, the same interrelationships exist in the smaller ones.

When a health worker becomes an employee, without being aware of the process, he will make some estimate as to the roles of the various members of the staff and as to who has the authority to make decisions. He will look for the individuals, health workers or professionals, who will be most helpful in his adaptation to a new field of work. At first, he will most likely react to what seems to be the negative aspects of the facility. With more experience some negatives will become positives. As he finds his place in the health care system and feels reasonably secure in it, he will have the time to look around him and try to see the patterns of operation, to begin to fit together the many parts of the entire health care system. Many changes in health care are in process, and he as a health worker will have to be flexible enough to change with them.

ASSIGNMENT: Everyone plays this game, so why don't you? Pretend you have the authority to make changes in the health care system—in your own work assignment, in the program of the facility in which you work. What changes would you make?

"Well, let's get on with it. . . ."

"'What do you think?'"

". . . if only there is someone near who cares. . . ."

"I know with my head. . . ."

"He's just a blank."

". . . a female Ben Casey. . . ."

". . . I felt as if I had failed Mrs. Purdy. . . ."

"To suffer and hurt with your patients. . . ."

"What a fool I've been."

10 the health worker's management of feeling

"We've talked about some of the ways patients and their families deal with illness, but what about you?" the author said thoughtfully.
The health worker approached this question with his usual caution. "Well, what about me?"
"How do you feel about working with sick people—about illness?"
"Why do you want to know?"
"Your feelings and attitudes are a part of patient care."
At his look of bewilderment and alarm, the author said gently, "It's never as easy to look at ourselves as it is to look at others, but it shouldn't be too bad. You've already learned more than you realize. . . ."
The health worker took a deep breath. "Well," he said, "let's get on with it. . . ."

intellectual response versus feeling response

A psychiatrist once said, "If I ask my patient 'What do you think?' I get an intellectual response which may or may not mean very much, but if I ask him how he feels about something, I get a gut response which is more likely to reveal the things he is troubled about."

The word "feeling" has been used frequently in this book. There have been discussions and examples of the ways patients have felt about health care and illness and how their families have felt, and there have been some examples of how the health worker has felt about his role and his experiences.

This chapter will be a more detailed discussion of feeling, particularly the health worker's. Why is feeling important? Because feeling, or emotion, is that part of the personality which gives it color and flavor and spice. Feeling is the most important ingredient in the relationship between two people.

Not only is feeling the most important thing, but it is also the first thing one looks for when meeting a person. Does he appear to be warm, friendly, outgoing, understanding; or does he seem to be cold, aloof, withdrawn, or negative? So accustomed are people to making this kind of assessment that they are often unaware that they are doing it, but not until such an assessment of feeling is made does one move to identify other characteristics which make one person different from all others.

At the same time, it's the feeling, or emotional, part of our personality which can sometimes get us into trouble. It is not what we think but how we feel which most often influences our actions. Such common expressions as these illustrate this point: "I know with my head what I should do, but my feelings make me do something else." "He always leads with his heart, rather than with his head." Or, "She lets her feelings run away with her." We are more apt to hear "He is emotionally ill" than "His thinking is confused." This latter statement usually indicates the influence of emotion upon thought. Thus, while the quality of feeling or emotion may enrich the personality, it may also lead to difficulties unless there is proper balance or control. To achieve balance one must first have some understanding of why one has a particular feeling or emotional response to a situation, and in order to discover why, one may have to look back upon his cultural background, his familial roots, or experiences which have profoundly influenced him. For anyone, but especially for the health worker, self-questioning may be a difficult and sometimes painful task, but yet a rewarding one. "Why do I feel this way?" he must ask himself and "How do my feelings influence the way I care for patients?" He will find it necessary to ask himself these questions not once but many times in the course of his career as a health worker.

lack of feeling

Since examples are often the best way to illustrate a concept, let us now look at some which indicate a lack of feeling, some which demonstrate too much feeling, and one in which there seemed to be a proper balance of feeling and action. The reader will recall the narrative of the patient in a mental hospital who had a frontal lobotomy.[1] This poignant story arouses pity, revulsion, and sadness in the reader and there is often anger that this kind of thing should have had to happen to any human being. Whatever the rationale for this surgery, these are people who were doomed for the rest of their lives to an existence in which they could never feel love or anger, pain or joy. How could they relate to anyone, or how could another person relate to them? This is an extreme example, but let us look at one which may have been equally as tragic, although not as spectacular. A nursing supervisor related this one.

withholding of feeling

He was a strange one. I never knew him, really, and I don't think anyone else did either. Nothing in his appearance was peculiar, hair a little too long but neat enough. A beard, but this is not unusual today. It was his eyes which troubled me. To myself, I thought of him as the boy with dead eyes. They were strange, pale blue. They might have been sightless for all the animation they

---

[1] Chap. 2, the section on origins of feelings and attitudes.

showed. Indeed, the boy's face gave little sign of any kind of emotion. As one of the staff said, "He's just a blank." And this is the way he appeared. I thought of drugs, but there was never any sign he had or was taking them.

He did his work well enough. He was quick to learn and never showed any reluctance to take on any task I assigned him. This was the surgical ward, and we had frequent emergencies. I could always count on his doing what I asked him to do, but he never volunteered. He would wait passively for orders. He never seemed to relate to anyone, staff or patients. I overheard two of the patients talking about him one day. "He gives me the creeps," one said and the other agreed. "He is kind of spooky; he comes into the room so quietly I don't know he's there if I have my eyes closed. You can't ever get him to talk to you. It's just 'yes, ma'am' and 'no, ma'am.' He's a funny one." The staff felt the same way. They tried to involve him. They invited him to coffee and would ask his opinion about things, but when he didn't respond, they just gave up and most of the time ignored him.

This bothered me. I tried to talk with him. "Do you like this work?" "Yes, ma'am." "Is there anything you don't like about it?" "No, ma'am." I said, "I don't feel I know you at all. I don't know how you feel or what you think. I am not trying to probe into your personal life—I have no right to do that. But I do like for the people on staff to feel free enough to ask questions or to talk about their job and how they would like to see things done. Most of the people around here speak their mind pretty freely. And I count on all the staff to help me understand the patients and let me know if anything is troubling them or if we are overlooking something they need. Do you understand what I am trying to say?" He just looked at me and said only, "Yes, I understand." I somehow felt he resented my effort to penetrate the wall he had built around himself, but I can't tell you how I sensed this. "I am not criticizing you," I said.

"Your work is all right. I am just interested in how you—in having you feel more comfortable with us." I stumbled around and didn't know how to put it and he didn't help me. He just said, *"Thank you ma'am,"* and went off.

Now that's the kind of interview which leaves a supervisor flat on her face. Nothing happened for the next few days. He went about his business as he always had. And then one morning he didn't show up for work. We never saw him again. He just seemed to have vanished. I always felt that if I hadn't tried to talk with him, he would have still been there. He, for reasons we will never know, seemed unable to have close relationships with anyone. What hurts he had sustained one can only speculate on, but I have often thought of him and wondered where he was and if anyone was ever able to reach him. But I must say that things went better on the ward after he left. He made everyone feel uncomfortable. A strange boy. A very strange boy.

The nursing supervisor continued:

I had another person on my staff for a while, a ward clerk, who concerned me, too. But while I felt only pity for the boy and, as I mentioned earlier, regret that I had been unsuccessful in relating to him, I ended up feeling anger at this young woman. She was a very pretty girl and very efficient. The charts were always up to date, the appointments always set up correctly. Messages were written out concisely and correctly. But as one of the medical students said ruefully after he had tried unsuccessfully to flirt with her, "She sure knows how to turn you off." This girl, too, did not relate to the rest of the staff. She went off on her coffee breaks with girls from other departments, which was all right, but she seemed to have no time for any small talk, the friendly give and take which was usually found in my unit. The rest of the staff soon learned to leave her strictly alone. We felt she didn't like any of us and in a subtle kind of way it seemed as if she disliked patients most of all. She was too polite to them, almost in an insulting kind of way. That sounds weird, doesn't it, but I would see a patient approach her desk smiling and then when this girl replied to her the patient would draw back as if she had been slapped. I tried talking with her also. She just looked at me blankly. "Isn't my work satisfactory?" she replied. "Yes and no. It's not so much what you do as how you do it. I am not happy about your relations with the other staff members, but I figure they can take care of themselves. With patients and their families, however, I expect every member of the staff to go out of their way to be warm and friendly." "But I don't understand. What have I said or done that is wrong?"

Before I could reply, I was called away on an emergency and I didn't have a chance to continue my conference for several days. In the meantime, it happened my husband and I dropped into a nightclub one evening and I saw this girl with a group near the front of the room. I almost failed to recognize her. She was laughing and talking animatedly, flirting with the man next to her. Anyone else seeing her would have thought what an attractive, charming young woman, but I felt anger. I didn't know which of the roles she had assumed was the real one, but I was quite sure she had known perfectly well what I had meant when I tried to talk with her.

The next day I talked with personnel and requested that she be transferred, recommending that it be to a department where there were no patient contacts. I told the girl my recommendations and I toyed with the thought of telling her I had seen her at the nightclub. But I didn't. It would not have done any good.

Some months later the head of the bookkeeping department said to me, "How did you ever come to give up this girl? She's a whiz. Never makes a mistake." "How does she get along with your staff?" I asked. He looked surprised.

"Why, I don't know, and I don't care as long as she does the work." "You can have her," I said.

too much feeling

Now to look at an example of a health worker who had too much feeling. In this instance a former nurse's aide describes an experience she once had.

When I first went to the nursing home I was just out of high school. I had some confused idea of being another "Lady with a Lamp," of patients responding to the gentle touch of my hand on their foreheads, or of being a female Ben Casey, gruff but with a kindly heart.

The reality of the nursing home was, of course quite different, but I didn't at first realize this. I found I really liked caring for some of the old people, the ones who could talk or knew what was going on. And I had my favorites. Mrs. Purdy was one of them. She reminded me of my Swedish grandmother who was a warm, loving woman, always joking and laughing. Although she was partially paralyzed, Mrs. Purdy could laugh at herself and at others. When she spilled her food, she'd say, "More work for you. I'm sorry." Then she'd make a face. "Helpless as a baby! Disgusting!" She didn't need anyone to tell her to try to help herself. She worked very hard at doing this.

She seemed to like my visits. Her face would light up when I came into the room. Sometimes she gave my hand a little pat.

One day I came to work and found that my Mrs. Purdy had had another stroke. This time she was almost completely immobilized. She could not speak. She had a little, very little, movement of her right hand. But I was positive she was aware and knew what had happened. Her eyes followed me as I changed her bedding and fluffed her pillows and got out a clean gown. As I did these things, I talked to her as I usually did of the happenings around the nursing home but I could hardly bear to look at her and see the anguish in her eyes. When other members of the staff came into her room, they acted and spoke as if she could no longer see or hear. "She knows what's going on," I insisted. "She understands everything you say." The nurse came by and I repeated my statement. She looked at Mrs. Purdy incuriously, "Maybe," she said and walked away.

I visited her when I could, but I have to say that I did not go into her room as often as I should have. The terrible pleading in her eyes got to me. But when I did go I would try to talk to her as I always had. I tried to think of things that might amuse her. Sometimes I would just hold her hand.

A few months after her second stroke I stopped at the door of her room, and I knew she had gone away, although she still breathed. It was as if shutters had been drawn over her eyes. There was no sign I could detect that she could any longer see or hear.

It was after her second stroke that I really faced the fact that no matter what I or anyone else did, all the patients in the nursing home were going to die and that some of them would get worse, as had Mrs. Purdy, before they did. I found myself wishing they all could die as my grandmother had, quickly, while they still knew what was happening, while they still were a part of life. These thoughts frightened me and I could not speak of them to anyone.

One morning a few months later when I arrived at the nursing home, I was told that Mrs. Purdy had died during the night. I turned around, walked out the door and never went back. For a long time afterward I felt as if I had failed Mrs. Purdy and all the other patients. It was not my first failure nor will it be my last one, but it hurt for a long time. . . .

As in all such narratives used to illustrate a point, these leave many unanswered questions. We can only speculate about the attendant who showed little emotion of any kind and apparently withdrew when friendly overtures were made to him as if any close relationship with another person frightened him. What the real story was, we will never know, but his isolation from the normal give and take of human relationships was a tragedy for him, and patients were deprived of something they needed very much.

The ward clerk! Which of her behaviors was the real one—the laughing, charming young woman in the nightclub or the coldly efficient young person who gave no outward sign of warmth or friendliness to the staff or the patients? Was she one of the people for whom work was "Just a job to be endured" or could her behavior possibly have masked some fear of involvement with sick people, of reaction to the human pressures and demands over and beyond the mechanics of a clerical job? We will never know.

The nursing supervisor agreed.

I've often thought of these two people. Perhaps because they both represent a failure on my part. If I had not pushed, but gone along on the attendant's terms, he might have eventually learned to trust me and relaxed a bit. Slowly he might have learned some small ways of sharing himself with other people. At some time in his life he must have been badly hurt. He wasn't born this way.

The ward clerk I didn't handle well because I was angry with her. So much potential for being a warm, giving person and yet so withholding—deliberately, I felt. Again, if I had waited and done some cautious exploration the ending might have been different. But you must remember that a supervisor always walks a tightrope. She has no right to venture into the personal lives of her workers unless they invite her. Even when their behavior affects their work, you can only move in a limited fashion. And you must never forget that your first responsibility is to the patients whose need for love is so great. Or, if "love" is too strong a word, whose need for "caring people" is so very

much a part of illness. How long can you wait for staff
people to take on the role? For assume it they must.

Too little feeling or too much. Both present problems for
the health worker and the patient. A social work supervisor
said:

> But I'll take the one with too much feeling any day.
> Sometimes they never get straightened out but usually as
> they gain in experience they learn how to manage their
> feelings, not to deny them, and they find that the emotion-
> al or feeling response is a valuable tool in learning about
> people and relating to them. The people—and there are
> some in health work—who see patients only as bugs stuck
> on the end of a pin never achieve understanding of people
> or gain good rapport with them. To suffer and hurt with
> your patients is a painful process, but it is one of the best
> ways I know of learning how to help them. I have a theory
> that unless health workers do go through this overexag-
> gerated state, they never amount to much.
>
> Your young girl in the nursing home really suffered from
> that experience, but she tells you the helpful and kind
> things she learned to do because of her feeling for her Mrs.
> Purdy: seeing her frequently, and after the second stroke,
> making herself go in, painful as it was; making herself do
> the little things that made the patient more comfortable;
> talking to her, treating her as a living person with feelings
> of anguish and pain. She felt that experience was a
> failure, but I am very sure she applied something of what
> she learned then to experiences she had later on. The sad
> thing for her is that apparently she found no one at the
> nursing home to whom she could talk, who would let her
> cry if necessary, but help support her until she could gain
> some perspective. We lose many people like this from the
> health field because we are too busy or don't have enough
> staff to help them through difficult experiences like this. It
> is very hard, especially on young workers.

the patient's need for love

The nursing supervisor said the patient's "need for love" or for "caring people" is a part of illness. When one is sick all emotions are accentuated: pain is exaggerated, fears are intensified, suspicions and angers are stronger, and the need for love—the desire to be cared for, to be protected—is often very strong. In the pages of this book there are many narratives describing how patients and their families deal with illness or injury, the things that are important when they are sick, their interaction with health workers and professionals. Patients have few, if any, criticisms of the technical aspects of their care. They seem to assume this is generally adequate or, if they do question it, they are reluctant to say so. However, in all the incidents described in these stories, one theme is repeated again and again and that is the patient's need for someone to treat him as a person—for someone to show him he cares about what is happening to him. This poignant plea is sometimes expressed but often revealed only in small, seemingly slight or insignificant comments or actions: the patient who said, "Don't take everything away that is me"[2] or the wife of the mental patient who was, in effect, saying to the young social worker, "Give me some crumb of understanding and sympathy. I feel so frightened and alone."[3] Another example was the Colonel's daughter who watched the door for the visitor who never came.[4] Still another illustration was the patient who made so many demands upon her physician.[5] She was actually trying to communicate her desperate need for understanding and acceptance. A patient not previously quoted in this book expressed his feeling in the following words: "All the indignities, all the pain I must experience, can be borne if only there is someone near who cares about me

[2]Chap. 2, the section on depersonalizing the patient.
[3]Chap. 7, the section on families' need for understanding.
[4]Chap. 7, the section on abandonment or desertion.
[5]Chap. 4, the section on listening.

and understands something of my fears and my loneliness. It doesn't really matter who it is, the doctor or the woman who scrubs the floor of my room. If only there is someone."

The needfulness of the patient and often of members of his family demands a response the health worker is not always able to make. The health worker may not know what to do. He may be afraid to take the required initiative, or his own needs for emotional support may be so great that he has little to give to anyone else.[6] The environment in which the health worker must practice, be it clinic, hospital, nursing home, research laboratory, or outreach health center, can bring to life some of his own fears about illness. In caring for the sick, these fears may increase.

management of feeling

Far too often the "caring" aspect of health service receives little attention or notice. Neither the patient nor the health worker gets much help in understanding his feelings or in learning how to manage them. And management it is, not denial of feeling but an honest recognition that certain situations and certain people create emotional reactions which may seem to be completely unreasonable and illogical but which have their roots in the experience and background of each person. Usually the patient and the health worker "muddle through" to some kind of resolution which may be good or bad.

origin of feelings

If, however, people can learn some method by which they can come to understand some of the reasons why they have particular feelings about certain events or people, they have

[6]The young social worker, Chap. 3, the section on feelings of dislike, or the nurse's aide in this chapter, the section on too much feeling, illustrates the not knowing, the fear, and the health worker's needs.

achieved the first step in the management of feeling. For the sensitive, introspective person, the method he uses may be just to sit down and reflect on the nature of his feelings and step by step to trace them back to their origins. For another person not accustomed or unable to use this technique, talking over his reactions with someone else may help him understand them better. For the health worker this someone may be a friend, a coworker, or a supervisor. If the feelings are so intense that they seriously interfere with his work, he may want to seek some kind of specialized help. For some health workers, withdrawing from the emotionally charged situation and seeking other employment may be the answer. Denial of feeling is never a satisfactory solution because it creates its own chain of reactions and the health worker may find himself in more difficulty rather than less.

Remember the often quoted lines from a song in the musical *South Pacific:*

"You've got to be taught before it's too late,
Before you are six, or seven, or eight."

It does seem that early experiences have great influence on shaping our attitudes, the way we feel, and how we express our feelings. In the field of health the worker brings certain attitudes and responses to illness and to patient care. As he gains in experience some of these may be modified, but not always. Sometimes the original attitudes may be strengthened and care for the patient is improved.

An example of the influence of early experiences on a health worker's performance was reported by her supervisor:

This young woman, a nurse's aide, had lost her mother when she was ten years old. Prior to her death, the mother, a cardiac patient, was a semi-invalid. However, she always made light of her illness, and exerted every effort to provide her children with a reasonably stable environment, encouraging them to go out to play, to have their friends in. A housekeeper was brought in to do the heavy work.

The daughter, no doubt influenced by her devotion to her mother, applied for work as a nurse's aide. She was unusually good with most patients—although she was inclined to do too much rather than too little for them. She was better with the independent patients who minimized their discomforts than with the dependent patients who complained a lot or those who were withdrawn and morose. She did not neglect any of them or express any dislike or irritation. She just seemed not as perceptive, as aware of how to help such patients. Sometimes she seemed quite bewildered by their behavior.

She was, however, a sensitive girl who learned quickly. When things did not go well between a patient and herself, she came and talked it over with me. And then she would go back and try again with her problem patient. She was not at first aware of the possible cause for her difficulties, and I did not push it, preferring that she discover it for herself. And she did. Rather shamefacedly, she remarked one day, "What a fool I've been. Here I have been expecting all my patients to handle their illness like my mother did. And when they didn't, I was disgusted and impatient with them. Why was I so blind?" I assured her that was how one's feelings could trap a person, and that it occurred quite frequently. She turned out to be one of my best health workers. When she got married and left for a job in another state, I was sorry for myself, although not for her.

In another quite similar situation, which also involved a nurse's aide, the problems were more complex. The nurse director described the situation in the following manner:

The father of this young woman had been an invalid as long as she could remember. He had rheumatoid arthritis and was often in pain and at times irritable. Her mother worked and when she was home she spent most of her time caring for her husband. The nurse's aide as a child had felt deprived of the normal amount of love and attention from her mother and she also was resentful that her father was never able to fulfill his role as a parent. She realized he couldn't help his illness, but she still had anger. I learned this quite by accident when one of her mother's friends, also a nurse, talked with me about her. I had been concerned about her ways with patients. She was inclined to be sharp and abrupt. She was critical when they complained of pain. "He's just putting it on" or "He just wants attention." She resented any of my efforts to talk with her about the way she responded to patients. I had thought of firing her, but when I found out about her childhood, I decided to keep on trying with her. It was not easy. She had many good qualities: worked hard, was willing to stay overtime when it was necessary, was quick and resourceful. Her relations with the rest of the staff were good. Eventually I was able to persuade her to get some counseling and she has turned out very well. But it took a while and there were times. . . .

Remember the patient in Chapter 7 whose mother was overly concerned about her children?[7] This patient's sister responded in exactly the opposite way to the mother's behavior. She denied, even when she really had need of a physician's care, that there was anything wrong with her. She always made quite a point of bragging about never having been ill in her entire life. Fortunately she did have better than average health. However, she was not very understanding or sympathetic when her husband or her children had any illness. It could well have been that underneath her denial was concern she never let herself face about illness. We will never know, because she died quite unexpectedly of a coronary.

SUMMARY: It is good to have the capacity to feel—even though the feeling or emotional part of one's personality may create problems if not handled properly. One of the best ways to manage feelings is to try to understand them and how they

[7]Chap. 7, the section on other problems.

came to be. Not easy and sometimes painful, but it can be done.

The environment in which the health worker grew up and the persons with whom he was most closely associated as a child will influence his attitudes toward health care and patients. Granny Sue's children raised on home remedies and taught to seek a doctor only at a time of crisis will have a different concept of medical care from someone raised in a ghetto or on a Minnesota wheat farm.[8] Granny Sue's rugged independence, even when dying, will be a model against which her children will measure the way other patients cope with illness and dying.

Only when he fully understands and controls his own emotions can the health worker be free to help meet his patients' needs. Only when he can appreciate and accept the fact that each patient's "need for love" is different from the next one's can he become a truly "caring person."

ASSIGNMENT: Think of two situations in which you felt you had too much or too little involvement with a patient. Try to identify the reasons for your reactions. How did you manage your feelings?

[8]Chap. 11, the section on influence of cultural patterns on patient attitudes.

"... worms under the carpet."

"... just a blob."

"... a cooperative patient."

"Doesn't anyone around here speak Spanish?"

"... Don't worry about a thing."

"... their ways of living and dying."

"I don't think this was one of our success cases."

"When her time came. . . ."

"... not having roots anywhere. . . ."

"It's scary. . . ."

11 what health worker and patient have in common

"You know what? I have just made a discovery," the health worker said, flopping down in the chair beside the author's desk. He was grinning.

"Indeed, tell me about it," the author said smiling back at him.

"I think the patients and the health workers should belong to the same union."

"A provocative statement. How did you arrive at that conclusion?"

"We both might just as well be worms under the carpet. No one in health care ever asks us what we think should be done about anything—and I mean anything. We both are told, 'Do this, or do that.' We have things done to us. But no one ever explains anything to us. No one even goes through the motions of asking what we think or how we feel."

"Those are pretty strong statements. Can you give me an example of what you mean?"

"Yes, I can," the health worker said emphatically. *"I have lots of them."*

common grievances of health worker and patient

The health worker's observation should be considered. Allowing for some bias on his part, there are some similarities between the status of patients and health workers. Patients have like reactions. They may also have their prejudices, but if both groups have similar feelings there must be some basis for them.

One of the examples the health worker gave was as follows:

They're remodeling the outpatient clinic. So down comes the chief of staff, who spends most of his time upstairs in a research lab, and the director of nursing, who fans through the clinic once in every six weeks, and the assistant administrator, who sometimes wanders in with a cup of coffee in his hand. But there they are with the architect and an armload of blueprints and they are busy. Yes, ma'am, they are busy, talking about what they are going to have done. The chief wants carpets everywhere. "It cuts down on the noise," he says, and maybe he's right, but they settle on the alcove for the waiting room. Now if they had asked me, I could have told them that that alcove always has a draft in the wintertime and no carpet is going to help that. Besides, it isn't big enough for all the patients we get in on a busy day.

But they don't ask me or anybody who works down there —not even the clinic nurse. They are deciding everything. And do you know what kind of chairs they are going to have? Those slick plastic jobs—the ones you slide around in and can't sit up straight in. Some of our old ladies crippled with rheumatism will have a bad time getting in and out of them. Wouldn't you think they'd know better—one of them at least? They've all had more schooling than I've had, but there they were arguing about colors and lamps.

There were patients sitting there. They could have asked them what they thought, even if they didn't want to ask one of us, but they didn't. They just stepped over and around them. . . .

The health worker got up from his chair and began

marching up and down the room as he always did when he was feeling strongly about something. Wheeling around he pointed his finger at the author and said sternly, "I have some more examples. Listen:

health worker's lack of identity

You talked about patients not being called by their names—well how many times do you think a health worker is called by his name? It's "Hey there, get this specimen to the lab," or "Will you take the cardiac in room 210 down to x-ray?" Most of us have name tags with print big enough for anyone not half-blind to read, but we could be here for ten years and have only a handful of people even know our name, much less call us by it. How do you think that makes us feel? Just like the patients—no identity—just a blob.

And another thing. Patients are always saying no one ever explains to them what is to be done to them or why. Well, health workers can gripe about this kind of thing too. If we could sometimes have someone explain to us why certain tests have to be done or why and how a blood sample is to be used. Oh, sure, I know what the answer is: everyone is too busy to take time to explain and then too the professionals probably wonder why we want to know. Well it isn't just nose trouble. It would make our jobs more interesting and, besides, some of us would like to learn while we are working. That "too busy" routine—well don't let them kid you. I don't mean a doctor has to stop in the middle of an operation or when he is taking care of a dying patient to talk to us, but there are plenty of times when they are drinking coffee back in the chart room or flirting with one of the nurses that they could spare us a few minutes.

Oh blast it all! I am just trying to say that if we felt more a part of what is going on, we'd like it better and I think we'd do better work, that old morale factor, you know. And

I also think that if somehow patients could be made to feel they had some say in what was being done to them—and if things were explained more to them—they would be— what's that word that is always being kicked around?—"a cooperative patient." Ha! I wonder if doctors and nurses and administrators ever give a thought to how they would run a health care program if they didn't have health workers to do most of the dirty work—and didn't have patients to work on?

patient's comments on being ignored

A patient in the same clinic to which the health worker was assigned was asked to read the above comments and give her opinions. A pleasant-faced, middle-aged woman who had had many illnesses, three or four hospitalizations, and was a frequent visitor to the clinic, she seemed well qualified to speak for patients. She smiled as she read the health worker's comments.

He's so right you know, although I don't know that I had ever thought about it in just that way. I think patients are so used to being "put down" that usually they just accept it. I don't mean they like it. No one wants to be treated as a "nothing," as if they were too stupid to understand or as if what they had to say was of no importance, but it happens so often. . . . I don't think the staff mean to mistreat us. Most of them are kind, nice people. It's just that they have so many things on their minds that they forget we have things on our minds, too. They also forget that most of the things they do are being done to us. I think patients would like to believe, or have someone pretend to help us believe, that we had something to say about the decisions which affect us. Why don't we speak up like the health worker does? Well, he's young. He's bright and knows how to express himself and he'll probably get some changes made. But patients . . . patients aren't as brave. If they do speak up they know they'll probably be ignored, or they run the danger of arousing anger. They are afraid to risk this. While they are a patient they have to depend on the health care staff to get them well. What if they are put out of the hospital or what if the doctor refuses to treat them? I don't know that this ever happens, but it's what patients are afraid of. The health worker can speak his mind and the worst thing that can happen to him is that he may get fired, but we have a lot more to lose.

What is almost funny, you know, is that we are braver after we are no longer a patient. We speak our minds then, not necessarily where it will do any good, but to our friends and our families. I remember once I tried to tell my doctor something I thought was important, and he interrupted me, "I'm the doctor. I know." Later when things didn't go right, he came charging into my room and said, "Why didn't you tell me about this?" I said I had tried to, but I don't think he believed me. . . . What can you do?

To go back to some of the things the health worker said. I had never thought that we had so many things in common—I am glad to know this. It will help me have a better understanding of health workers and to be more tolerant of some of the things they do. It's kind of a pecking order isn't it? The health workers get stepped on or ignored and they in turn sometimes take it out on patients. The only thing is, patients have no one lower than they are on whom to vent their frustrations—unless it's their families.

I'll say a word about the health worker's comments about the clinic redecorating, and then I am going to stop. This is a minor part of patient care—but it's a good example of how we are treated. Yet, who spends more time in a clinic than the patients? We have a lot of opportunity while we are playing the "waiting game" (that's what the patients call the hours we sometimes spend in the clinics) to do a lot of thinking about how things could be improved. I think patients—and yes, health workers too—could have a lot to contribute to how a clinic is arranged and planned. In this clinic pretty curtains and a carpet would brighten up the place and goodness knows it needs it. But I think the most important thing is a comfortable chair. When you don't feel well, a good chair can be very soothing. I overheard talk about piping music into the waiting room. Well, I don't mind, but I know some of the patients don't like this idea. If they have a headache or are feeling down in the dumps, they say music makes them feel worse, but I guess the top people never think of things like that.

effect of negative experiences on patient and health worker

The health worker has strong feelings about being ignored, about losing his identity, and about feeling of little worth, and these things merit such reactions. The patient also has much expressed and unexpressed anger at the loss of dignity—the assaults upon his self-image. This is an area in which much work needs to be done for both patient and health worker. The patient who feels respected as a person—who feels he is liked or even loved by the people who care for him—can endure many indignities and much pain. It is equally true that the health worker, if his self-image is supported and he is able to maintain pride in himself, can do remarkable things in his role as a member—an important member—of the health care team. Now, far too often both patients and health workers feel as if they have little power to effect any change in their present status.

These feelings of the health worker and of the patient may account for some of the dissatisfaction both within and outside the health care system. Much of this is not directly expressed and is probably not even recognized by either the health worker or the patient. The patient expresses his anger or resentment by such comments as, "I have to wait so long when I go to the clinic," "My doctor is too busy to give me much time," "Everything is so impersonal." The health worker is apt to project his anger upon the working conditions, the long hours, or the unreasonable demands made upon him.

positive elements shared by health worker and patient

There is, however, a positive aspect to this negative situation; this is that both health worker and patient have so many things in common, not only bad but good experiences. Awareness of this fact could well be the first step in developing good interpersonal relations between the two of them and might in turn produce some changes in the health care system.

Some of the negative experiences shared by the patient and health worker have been described, but now let us look at some of the positives. Many patients and health workers share the same cultural, racial, and economic background. It is not unusual for the health worker to be from the same small town, same neighborhood, or same ghetto area as the patient. He, better than anyone else in the health care system, knows the patient and is more likely to make an accurate assessment of how the latter feels—what he needs.

The fact, however, that the health worker might have this kind of knowledge and could make a valuable contribution to the care and treatment of the patient usually goes unnoticed. For most patients too little use is made of the information about his racial or cultural background. These facts are not identified as significant. Sometimes it takes a crisis to call attention to them, and once the crisis is past their value is quickly forgotten. Even though the health worker has made a valuable contribution to patient care, it is likely to receive little attention.

contribution of health worker to patient care

An example is the elderly woman struck by a car and brought into the emergency room of the city hospital by the police. She apparently had a broken hip and minor bruises and injuries.

She seemed frightened, confused, and in pain, but no one could get any information from her because she could not speak English. From the few words she uttered it was thought she was Mexican or of Spanish origin.

"Doesn't anyone around here speak Spanish?" asked the orthopedic surgeon who had been called in to examine her. No one did—none of the nurses, medical students, or interns.

The surgeon was irritated. "Don't we have anyone in the hospital who does? Well find out. Call the social service department. Go out on the street and drag someone in who does, if you have to. I don't like doing surgery until we know something about her. She's so scared." He patted the patient on the shoulder and made reassuring gestures, but she still appeared terrified.

The social service department had no one who could speak Spanish, but the social worker got in touch with the police, found out where the patient had been struck by the car, and located the nearest church. There she learned that the priest, Father Gonzales, was out in the parish but was expected back shortly. She left word for him to call her. Rather pleased with herself, she reported what she had done to the surgeon.

He was not as happy as she had thought he would be. "Well and good, but that could take two or three hours. I can't wait that long."

The head nurse called personnel. She was told that their records did not contain information about the languages the personnel could speak; however, they thought they had two or three Mexican employees. They would try to locate one of them. In a short while they reported back that Luis Mūnos, a laboratory technician in pathology, could speak Spanish and was on his way down to the emergency room. When he appeared, he approached the surgeon hesitantly. No one had explained why he was wanted.

"I understand you speak Spanish," the surgeon said.

Luis nodded.

"Come with me. We have a patient whom we think is Mexican. I want you to talk with her. She doesn't understand us and we don't understand her." He led the way into the patient's room, followed by the nurse and a couple of medical students.

At Luis's first words, the old woman burst into tears and clutched his hand. Then she spoke rapidly, gesturing toward the doctors and toward her hip.

"She wants to know when she can go home and can something be done for the pain."

"Tell her we think her hip is broken, but we have to x-ray. If it is we will have to set it. She should stay here for a day or two, even if it isn't broken, to be sure nothing else is wrong. If it is broken, it will be a few weeks. Now be sure she understands all this—and yes, we will give her something for the pain."

The old woman began to weep again when Luis talked to her. *"She says her husband is old and sick and needs her."*

The surgeon ran his fingers through his hair. *"Tell her we will see what can be done about him. God knows what,"* he added parenthetically. *"But we must take care of her first. Tell her we will do something,"* he said firmly to Luis. *"Just get her name and address and find out if she's been to any other hospital. We will let everything else wait till she feels better, but tell her everything will be all right. Not to worry about a thing."*

At about this point, the priest arrived. Yes, Maria Esposito was one of his parishioners. He would see about the husband. While he was talking, Luis slipped away and no one noticed he was gone.

The next morning, when the surgeon made rounds with his staff, he found Maria pale but smiling. She tried to talk, but neither the surgeon nor his staff knew what she was saying.

"Where's that boy—that lab technician?" asked the surgeon impatiently.

"I'll get him," the head nurse said.

As she turned away, he asked, "Did anyone thank him for help us out yesterday?" No one had. "Well, neither did I and if we hadn't needed him again I guess I would never have thought of it."

When Luis came and talked with Maria Esposito, he translated her words for the staff. "She says she wants her rosary. Someone took it away yesterday and she has never been parted from it since the priest gave it to her as a little girl. And," he hesitated, "she is not happy with the food. It has no taste." He turned to Maria Esposito as if to confirm this statement and she nodded and made a face.

"The rosary she can have. It is in the safe," the surgeon said. He smiled ruefully. "The food. We all gripe about the food, but I am not sure I am brave enough to tackle the dietician. What do you think I should do, Luis?"

"If it would be all right, we could bring in some of her kind of food."

"Oh, dear," the nurse said. "We try to discourage relatives bringing in food to the patients."

"True, but in this case," the surgeon said, "she must eat and get the right nourishment if her bones are to knit properly." He told Luis, "The hospital food may not taste good, but it has the things she needs. If she will try to eat it, you can bring in some tortillas or whatever she wants." Luis repeated this remark to the patient and she made another face but nodded assent. As he turned to leave the room, the surgeon said, "Tell Maria she is doing great. And, oh, yes, can you drop by my office after rounds are over?"

When Luis came to the office, the surgeon thanked him for his help and told him, "While Maria is in the hospital, I want you to drop by and see her every day. If she needs something or doesn't understand anything, let the head nurse know. I would like for you to act as an interpreter and explain to her the things we need to know and also to help her understand what we are doing and why. Can you do this? I will talk to your lab chief and get his permission so you won't get into any trouble."

"We Chicanos usually do this anyway. When one of our people come into the hospital, we see them and take messages back and forth to their families. Or run errands for them."

The surgeon leaned back in his chair and looked at him. "You mean all that work trying to find someone yesterday wasn't necessary?"

"Oh, no! That was an emergency. She was very frightened and needed someone right away."

"But if anyone had known about you, it would have saved some time. With some patients. . . ."

"True. I am sorry. Word was slow getting to us about her."

"How many employees do we have who speak Spanish?" Luis shrugged. "Quite a few."

"Do you know anyone in the hospital who speaks Indian— American Indian?"

Luis smiled. "Yes."

"And Italian?"

"Perhaps."

"I will remember that."

Later the surgeon said to his staff, "I wonder how many things go on around this place we know nothing about." He turned to the head nurse, "Let's see if personnel can't run through the employee list and check out the language item. And we need to have such information where we can get to it quickly."

One of the interns spoke up. "Maybe some of us should learn a language."

The surgeon looked at him thoughtfully. "I wonder what Luis would say to that?"

"I know," a medical student said smugly. "I asked him. He was polite. It would be helpful, he said, but just learning a language wouldn't teach us the important things—about people's fears and hopes, their ways of living and dying."

The resident looked bewildered. "How do you learn those things?"

"Maybe," another resident said, "we ought to have Luis and his friends set up a seminar for us."

"Maybe Luis ought to sit in on some of our staff meetings," the medical student suggested. . . .

value of cultural patterns

A seminar might be helpful—or better still a series of seminars stressing the value of knowing and utilizing cultural patterns in the treatment of patients. Having health workers sit in on staff meetings is not a new idea. This has been done, particularly in psychiatric hospitals where the concept of the therapeutic community is practiced. Sometimes the role of the health worker is clearly defined, but often the reason for inviting them is to teach rather than learn from them. Both objectives have value.

Luis has much to teach the staff about Maria Esposito. The hospital is a strange environment for her. Many things understood or taken for granted by other patients may puzzle and frighten her. When she is ready for discharge Luis can tell them where and how she lives. Whether she will have to struggle up two or three flights of stairs to a cold water flat. Whether there is anyone who can help her. Does her husband need any medical care? Will she be able to return to the hospital for physical therapy? Questions which, if she spoke English, might be asked by another member of the staff and answered by her, but whether she would speak freely to someone of another culture about her real concerns, her beliefs (and superstitions), her desires, is another question. It is too often assumed that, if an individual feels only goodwill and has only good intentions, that whoever he is talking to will sense this and respond, but what cannot be known is what a lifetime of experience may have taught the individual about trust and the sharing of innermost feelings with a stranger.

Now to return to Maria Esposito. "Why do we need to know these kinds of things about her?" someone on the staff is sure to ask. "She's not a psycho. She just has a fractured hip." How does one know what she is and what she needs? Let her not be dismissed too quickly as "the fracture in room 305." Luis and his friends can teach the other members of the staff many things they do not know, but a great deal will depend upon the kind of communication that evolves among them.

example of poor interpersonal relations

In the following example there was no Luis—or if there was he did not come forward and identify himself—and no one thought to seek him out. Little Mary Tallchief, a two-year-old Indian baby was flown to the city hospital from a reservation. She was critically ill with pneumonia. A Public Health nurse had arranged for her admission and brought her in. The pediatric nurse described what happened:

It was one of those cases where everything goes wrong. At first, all our efforts were directed toward getting the baby through the crisis in her illness. Then we found we had a lot of questions and no answers. The medical history was incomplete and no one was certain whether the Public Health nurse had been unable to supply all the essential information or whether the resident had failed to put it all down. All we knew of the parents were their names and that they lived on a reservation in a remote part of the state. The address proved to be incomplete, and we didn't know how to reach them. The nurse had gone to another reservation and we couldn't locate her. Oh, it was a mess! We didn't know whether the baby had been abandoned— or what had happened. All we knew was she was very, very sick—and none of us knew how to communicate with her.

I can't remember all the details—but I do recall that after about a week we discovered that the mother was living within three blocks of the hospital. She was staying with a relative, but was apparently too shy and frightened to come to the hospital. How she got to the city from the reservation we never knew. The social worker went out and brought her to the hospital and when she was united with her baby—well—we knew it had not been abandoned. She held it so tightly we were almost afraid she would smother it. How do you describe scenes like that? I don't know. Anyway we were afraid she would just walk out of the hospital with the child—and it was still very ill—but she didn't. She spoke some English—although we never were sure just how much she understood. We couldn't get much history from her. She would just nod or shake her head or just look at us. We tried everything we could think of, but we never felt she trusted us or got over being afraid someone would snatch her baby away from her again. I will never understand how the Public Health nurse or anyone else was able to separate the two of them at the time the baby was brought to the hospital. True, little Mary was very ill and needed hospitalization, but I will always wonder—why didn't the mother come with her? They both needed each other so much.

We put a cot in the child's room. The mother's meals were brought in on a tray. She watched everything that was done for the baby—but did not interfere. "But she kind of scares me," the student nurse said. "She sits on the edge of her chair as if she is ready to spring at anyone she thought was hurting her baby." As the child improved, the mother seemed to relax a little, but she still did not respond to the staff's overtures.

At the time of discharge, we urged the mother to be sure and bring the baby back to us if she got sick again, but she made no response. The social worker offered to help her get back to the reservation, but the relative who up until now had uttered hardly a word, spoke up. "We take care of our people," he said, and that was that. They went off and the student nurse who watched them until they turned the corner of the corridor said tearfully, "I don't think this was one of our success cases."

This narrative leaves many unanswered questions. Why didn't the mother accompany the baby to the hospital? There may have been a good reason why she did not, but this should have been known. The hospital staff meant well, but they performed poorly in interpersonal relations. Somewhere in that city there must have been someone who could have helped both the mother and the staff achieve better understanding. It is even possible some of the health workers were Indian or of Indian descent. Although the baby recovered from its illness, if it should become ill again will it ever be possible to persuade the mother to take it to a doctor or to another hospital?

influence of cultural patterns on patient attitudes

There are isolated pockets—small remote communities—where life goes on as it has for several generations. The Indian reservations are one example, the Southern highlands are another. In the cities we still find small close-knit communities of one or another racial group, the Puerto Ricans, the Cubans, the blacks lately come from the deep South, older communities still predominantly Italian or Polish in background. All racial groups or combinations of them are to be found somewhere in this country, each with a mingling of old and new ideas about health care—folk medicine, voodoo medicine, faith healing. All of these and many others may influence patients' attitudes about accepting and receiving modern methods of treatment. Many patients, for example, are deeply mistrustful of hospitals "where they experiment on people." Others cling to the old ways because they are the known and familiar. Granny Sue was one of these:

When her time came, the word went out and her relatives gathered in her one-room cabin to wait until death arrived. The young doctor who had been called in was

*horrified when he saw so many people in one small room.
"Clear out, all of you!" he ordered, "you're using up all the
oxygen."
But Granny Sue, even on her deathbed, was in control of
her environment.
"I want them here," she croaked.
"Well, it's your funer—business!" the young doctor snapped
and left.
The relatives brought in food and drink and when Granny
Sue died, they gave her a proper funeral before dispersing.
There were no tears. Death was a part of life.*

Granny Sue had ordered the manner of her dying as she
had ordered the way of her life. Fortunate Granny Sue! Many
people become ill or die far from the place of their origin.
Others have no roots and the ties to their families were never
the close interlocking relationships Granny Sue maintained
with her kinfolk and especially with her children. In her small
community most of the people were related to her—and
everyone knew everyone else.

It is Granny Sue's children, however, who are caught with
one foot rooted in the past and one in the present. She
"birthed" twelve children in that one-room cabin, most of
them with the aid of a midwife. The doctor was called in only if
something went wrong. Of those still living, only two remain
near their birthplace. The others are scattered over the country. One, a career soldier, is on overseas duty. Another is a
factory worker in Detroit. A daughter lives in a housing project
in New York City with her two children and her mother-in-law,
who is blind. She works in the admitting office of a city
hospital! She says:

*People don't live in one place all their lives like they used
to. Now they move around a lot more. Sometimes it's
because they get married, like I did, or it's a job—or it's
just the way things are now. But sometimes you get a
queer kind of feeling—when you think about not having
roots anywhere and you know your kids won't either. My*

mother-in-law is always telling them stories about where she lived when she was young—poor kids they don't know that most of the stories are for real—they've never seen a live cow, or a pig, or run through grass in the country barefooted. My mother-in-law is eating her heart out because she wants to go back where she came from—but she doesn't know it's not like it was when she left it some fifty years ago. I listen to her, and some of the things she talks about I remember too. Sometimes I think, would I like to go back to live where I was born—but I know now that Ma is dead there's nothing there for me or my kids. Everything is changed. Most of the young people have left and don't come back—like me.

At work—at the hospital—I can tell right away the ones who have come from the country—from places like I lived in. Sometimes it is the way they dress or the words they use like "puny," "ailing," "feeling porely," but it is mostly the way they act. People who come from my part of the country are very proud. They are more ashamed at not having much education than anything else. Having kids without a father, or a husband in jail—they will tell you that—but they don't like to say if they don't have much education. And if they don't know something—they won't tell you. If one of the doctors talks to them and uses some fancy words—and then asks if they understand, they most always say, "Yes, of course." Then they go look up someone like me and ask what he meant. I don't know lots of times, but have been here long enough so I know where to go to find out. My kind of people are proud about taking help of any kind. They are like my Ma, who was used to doing for herself. I have seen some patients walk out of the doctor's office with a handful of prescriptions and tear them up—when they didn't have money to pay for them.

Trying to find a place for themselves in a city—to live, to work, to go to church—is hard for people like me who come from places where everything is known—the people, the land—what to expect and what to count on. It's scary—trying to live in a city and if you get sick it's worse. Back home, my Ma always knew some kind of home remedy for most of the things that ailed us—if she didn't there was the doctor to go to. He had been there a long time—and most of us knew him. If we didn't have the money to pay him, he took care of us anyway. Here, unless you have a lot of money or have lived here a long time and know where to go, you have to use a clinic or hospital. They are so big and so crowded, it's hard to find your way around. And no one seems to have that kind of "caring for people" that I grew up with.

I worry about if I would get sick. What would happen to my kids—or my mother-in-law? I suppose some of my family would come and take the children—and she, my mother-in-law, would be put in a nursing home. She wouldn't live long in one of those places. Working here, I know more about what to expect if I would come here as a patient—but it still would be scary. Most country people are afraid when they come here—but they don't want anyone to know they are. . . .

Yes, the "hill people" are proud and slow to trust strangers. "I have lived in this community for forty years," an elderly physician said, "and people still consider me an 'outlander' because I wasn't born and raised here." Luis will tell you the Chicanos are equally proud. The Indians, each tribe with its complex system of ritual and social structure, are also slow to share their real feelings with people outside their group. The blacks too have their own cultural patterns. Sometimes they are the most adept at seeming to take on the manners and values of white Americans, and yet at the same time the most articulate at defining the areas in which their ideologies clash with other groups.

There is great temptation to describe in much greater detail the influence of the cultural background upon the patient and the health worker and how these affect their adjustment to the health care system—either as patient or as worker. Here, however, the concern is the contribution the health worker can make to patient care because they both may have a common origin. This area is not well defined. Often it is not even identified by either the professional or the health worker. The usual pattern for both groups is training only in the techniques of their work, leaving the "human element" under which the cultural background is included to be discovered on an individual basis, often quite by accident or not at all. How can this situation be changed? First, there must be recognition of the value of knowing and understanding a patient's background and utilizing this knowledge in his treatment. Ideally, this recognition should come from the administrative or educational division of a health care unit. Material about this aspect of patient care should be included in all training courses for both the professional and nonprofessional.

Realistically, such programs as these are rare. If they are given, it is only in large teaching hospitals. Sometimes even in such places there is only a lecture or two on the cultural background—sketched only in broad general terms—not specifically related to the everyday care and treatment of patients. The contribution of the health worker is ignored.

a new role for the health worker

If the personnel department kept more detailed records on the health worker's background—the area in which he was born and raised—and the languages he spoke, this might be useful when emergencies arose—such as the one in which Luis was helpful. But this data would be of little value unless the staff were aware of the importance of such information and actually used it. Another hindrance to the effectiveness of such material is found in the health worker's own attitude. Often, like the patient, he is ashamed of his background and will frequently conceal it—by changing his name, by failing to give details about his actual place of birth or nationality. For example, few Indians will say they were born on a reservation. They give the name of the nearest town to the reservation as their place of birth.

If the health worker's knowledge is to be properly used in the care and treatment of patients, he will have to give accurate information. He must in some way regain his pride in his place of origin—in his racial ties. And he will in most cases have to take the initiative in letting the rest of the health care staff know he can be of aid in helping them understand some of the needs of patients which seem related to his background. He, the health worker, will have to be ingenious in doing this— extremely sensitive—and tactful. He may quietly say, "I can speak Spanish. If it would help I can speak with the patient and maybe help her not to be afraid of talking to you," or "The patient isn't angry—she is scared and doesn't understand what you are saying, but she doesn't like for you to know her English is not so good." There will be many failures and rebuffs, but if the health worker can develop a pride in himself and under- stand the importance of this kind of contribution to patient care, he should be a much more valuable employee and a happier one. There is no doubt but that there is "under- ground" communication between the health worker and pa- tient, but this has its limitations. If it is identified as a worthy and useful function, it can be utilized in many ways, not only in times of crisis but in many everyday tasks.

SUMMARY: This chapter discusses the health worker's dis- covery that he and the patient have much in common. Some of the negatives both experience are identified. The positive elements which the two frequently share—a common heritage and environment—are also noted. This bond may lead to good communication between the patient and health worker. It is of greater importance, however, that this positive interaction can improve patient care. Ideally, recognition of this potential should come from the educational or administrative arm of the health care system. If it does not, the health worker may have to take the initiative, acting as the link between the patient and the rest of the health care staff, interpreting his needs, his fears, and thereby helping him to understand the strange world of health care. In addition to improving patient care, this role should also enhance the self-esteem of the health worker. This function is often fraught with frustrations and will require much imagination and creativity from the health worker as well as personal courage.

ASSIGNMENT: Take two or three patients whom you know best and identify the positive and negative elements you share with them. Also describe what you might do as a liaison person between the patient and the staff.

4 learnable skills

"... aren't there any rules or guidelines ...?"

"... the 'little things' ... are really just good manners."

"I used to worry just about myself. ..."

"... like having a built-in antenna. ..."

"... 'Hang in there, kid. ...'"

"... keep your cool. ..."

"You know I'm hooked. ..."

"'Wrong room, Charlie. ...'"

"... don't try to play God. ..."

"You must walk alone."

12 some guidelines for the health worker

The health worker came into the author's room and without speaking sat down beside the desk. He seemed preoccupied and was frowning slightly. Still not speaking, he got up and walked up and down the room. Then he returned to his chair and sat down again.

"See here," he began, "in this business of learning about patients—and ourselves," he added hastily when the author made a slight movement, "aren't there any rules or guidelines we can use?"

The author looked doubtful, "You know how strongly I feel about trying to fit human behavior into any kind of an $a + b = c$ schedule."

The health worker grinned, "I ought to," then he grew serious. "I think I am just trying to find a way to put down in some kind of order some of the things I have learned about patient interaction. I can't think of what to call it or just how to do it. Maybe I am looking for some guidelines, something I can go back to every now and then when I get stuck. . . ." He shrugged, "I just don't know. . . ."

"Would it help if we made a list of the elements or precepts we have found to be important in our relations with patients?"

"Maybe, but first I want to see how you present them."

principles, precepts, or elements

These elements can be considered as the foundation of good human relations, whether with the sick or the well, with parent or child, with friend or enemy. However, this discussion will be limited to relations with patients. Further knowledge and experience may lead the health worker to make some modifications or additions, but this should be a good, basic list of "ground rules" to which he may refer until they become so much a part of him that they are utilized without awareness or plan. Included in this listing is some discussion of poor and good application of the various guidelines, but the health worker should be able to cite other examples which will have greater significance because they derive from his own learning.

respect

We talk of treating the patient with respect, but no precept is violated more often. Some of the violations are the fault of the health care institution. Examples of these are the long periods of waiting, the complex business office regulations, or demeaning admission procedures. If, however, the health worker must communicate some of the institution's requirements, the manner in which he does it is his responsibility. If he is haughty, officious, hostile, or indifferent, he is showing little regard for the patient.

When a health worker enters a patient's room without knocking, fails to introduce himself, does not explain why he is there, or does not address the patient by his name, he is showing little consideration for the patient. The failure to offer some small courtesy, such as lowering a shade, moving a table within reach of the patient, or arranging the pillows to make him more comfortable, or a delay in answering a bell is an affront. When two health workers chat about their own affairs while they perform some task for the patient, such as change his bed linens or wheel him down to physical therapy—in effect treat him as if he had no sight or hearing—these actions demonstrate little appreciation of the patient as a person. If he is aware of these insults, successful interaction may never be possible. Patients are often removed from their normal channels of communication, from their usual pattern of living, from their family and friends, and this isolation often tends to make them supersensitive to slights, real or imaginary.

The health worker thought about these comments:

"These are the 'little things' you are always talking about," he said thoughtfully. *"If they are done properly they are really just good manners. The kind of things you should do with anyone, sick or well. I guess you are right, though. These kinds of things are the ones that are always getting overlooked. I think I am going to remember them, but when I get in a hurry. . . . Take yesterday, for instance. When I walked into the lab, there were three orders waiting for me—every one marked Stat—and all of them in different parts of the hospital. I dash up to the room of a patient just admitted and I do all the things you have just mentioned. I don't knock. I just mumble something, grab her arm, and jab a needle into it. Halfway out of the door I look back, and she is just sitting there, staring at me, looking half-mad and half-frightened and lost. I know I ought to go back and apologize, but I don't. I keep on going. With the next patient, I do a little better and we get along just fine, but I walk out of his room and the nurse shoves three more orders at me and I take off—forgetting to do everything but the blood samples. I wonder,"* he concluded gloomily, *"if I will ever learn?"*

"I think you will. Once you would not have given a thought to how a patient should be treated."

"You are right about that," the health worker sighed. *"I used to worry just about myself, whether I'd get fired—or do some dumb thing and have everyone laughing at me—now. . . . Well what do you have for the next one?"*

awareness

Awareness is the quality of being conscious of the patient's state of wellness or illness, of noting marked changes in his condition. The changes in condition might be physical—pronounced difficulty in breathing, restlessness, or a change in skin color—or it might be a behavioral change. A patient, ordinarily friendly and responsive, is sullen and uncommunicative. Another patient, usually quiet and unassuming, is talkative and excited.

Awareness means sensitivity to the special kind of caring the patient needs. Does he want conversation, or does he want the health worker to move quietly and speak softly? Does he need some special assurance he is not alone, showing this by clinging to the health worker's hand? If the patient is a child, nothing may be of more comfort than to be held for a few minutes in the health worker's arms. Every patient will have some particular need which he may indicate by what he says or, more often, by what he doesn't say, by the way he sits or lies in bed, by the tone of his voice, rather than by the words he uses. This precept demands not only a high degree of perception from the health worker but also the ability to make a quick estimate of a situation and to act upon it.

The health worker nodded his head slowly.

"Yes, this is a rough one. I suppose it's like having a built-in antenna which tunes in on what the patient is trying to tell you, even though the patient doesn't use any words. But the thing that scares you is that it's so easy to read the messages wrong. Like when you walk into a patient's room and find her all smiles and making jokes and if you don't take the time to look more closely you don't see that she's clenching and unclenching her fists, that her voice is near to breaking, and that at any moment she is going to climb the wall from sheer fright or desperation. That's what shakes me up—nearly missing something like that. And deciding what is the best thing to do also can undo you. With that girl I just patted her on the shoulder

and said, 'Hang in there, kid,' and then I went for the nurse.

"*I remember another near miss. This was a real lady, always very polite and pleasant. Well, one day I went into her room to take her temperature and I thought she was asleep. I decided I would come back for her temperature a little later because she had been sleeping badly and I thought she could do with a little rest. But just as I was easing myself out of the room I heard a kind of whimper and I realized she wasn't asleep but was crying very quietly as if she didn't want anyone to hear her. Me, I never know what to do about a woman's crying, so I go for the nurse again. But I am curious as to what she will do, so I watch from the doorway. She just walks in and sits down by the bedside and takes the patient's hand in hers and pats it. 'What's the matter, my dear?' she says very softly. The patient doesn't answer at first because she is crying so hard. The nurse doesn't say anything but just sits there holding her hand until she is calmer and then she gets her to tell her what is wrong. I had to leave, but the nurse told me later she stayed until the patient fell asleep.*"

"*You seem to have a good understanding of this principle,*" *the author commented,* "*and you are learning to identify problem situations, but what are you going to do about them when there isn't a nurse or anyone else around? You are going to have to learn this too, you know.*"

The health worker didn't reply. He just nodded.

acceptance

Acceptance means acknowledging and responding to the patient's image of himself. It also means acceptance of the patient's ways, interfering only when he may be of harm to himself or others. It's acceptance of his ways of thinking, of his ways of believing or not believing, even though these are not your ways.

In small ways, in small things, the patient learns whether the health care staff accepts him or not. In one nursing home, the elderly patient found his only comfort in the chewing tobacco his friends smuggled in to him. He thought the staff was unaware of his habit, but one day an elderly nurse walked in and caught him. "She didn't say a blasted word," he confided to his cronies later. "She just sniffed and marched out of the room, but ever since then the whole staff acts as if I had smallpox. They don't say anything, it would be better if they did, but I get the message. Chewing tobacco is a filthy, dirty habit, and no one but a bum would use it. To Hell with them," he ended defiantly.

A visiting nurse recalled her shocked surprise when one of her Italian patients swore at her children.

She was a truly beautiful woman, which seemed somehow to make it all the more surprising. She had quite a vocabulary. I was horrified and I know I showed it. My impulse was to snatch up those poor little children and spirit them away to a saner and more respectable environment, but young as I was I realized that was not realistic. My next impulse was to scold her for talking to her children like that, but I must confess I was a little intimidated by her. Then I noticed a curious thing. The children weren't the least afraid of her. They stayed well out of arm's reach, but I had a suspicion they were proud of her performance. In fact I think they egged her on. And within minutes after that outburst, they were swarming all over her and she was hugging and kissing them. Even to my inexperienced eyes there was no doubt of the love and affection between them. The words didn't matter. . . .

It has often been remarked that most wars have been and are still being fought in the names of religion or politics. The pioneers in the early days of the West knew this. No one ever asked a stranger his name; it was "What do you call yourself, partner?" Nor was the stranger queried as to his religion or his politics. Whatever he volunteered about these subjects was accepted without comment. The men of the West had learned that many a bloody fight had erupted when two people disagreed about one of these subjects. Recently a plush retirement home was thrown into an uproar because one of the elderly ladies criticized what the minister had said in the morning prayer. Throughout that day and probably for days to come residents discussed the matter and took sides. "Did you hear what Margaret Duff said to the minister this morning? Wasn't it a disgrace?" "Of course not. She had a perfect right to disagree and to say so." People who are deeply religious sometimes find it very difficult to accept the fact that some people have different beliefs and others none at all. If religion is very important to the health worker—and it is to many of them—this may be an especially difficult area. Not to impose one's own beliefs on the patient and to accept the fact that he has a right to his own belief or nonbelief may require much self-control. It is equally important that the health worker never make light of the patient's beliefs no matter how strange they may seem.

The health worker seemed more comfortable with this principle.

"This one isn't as hard as the others. People are different. They'll act differently. They'll think differently. So you keep your cool and don't get into a sweat about it."

"Good. I think you do quite well in this area most of the time. I have only one concern. I sometimes seem to sense some irritation or impatience when people don't think as quickly as you do, or act as rapidly as you do. I am aware of this with staff more often than with patients."

"If something has to be done, I feel, well let's do it and get it over with."

"A very good attitude, but everyone doesn't think as quickly as you do or move as rapidly. To hand your own words back to you, 'People are different.'"

"Well I—you are right, I'll have to watch that."

concern

"I have a concern," the Quakers used to say when they went to the aid of a less fortunate neighbor. Concern is the feeling part—the caring—that we have for patients. The major emphasis of this book has been on this aspect of health care. It must be remembered that *feeling cannot be taught,* but if one has the capacity to reach out to others, to have compassion, to have empathy, to care, then *feeling can be trained* so it does not spill out indiscriminately, obscuring reason and judgment. It is the most effective element in the communication between two people. Spoken or unspoken, it's the feeling we look for when we meet a stranger. It's the capacity for feeling we assess when developing a friendship or seeking a marriage partner.

Young health workers in their eagerness to be professional often interpret a show of feeling as unprofessional behavior. Only when they have experience and are sure of themselves can they show emotion. A display of emotion must have certain controls, however, if it is to be appropriate. The adult who indulges in infantile temper tantrums is an example of a person who is poorly managing his feelings. To show concern and feeling, but not to overload the patient and not to let feeling control care, should be the objective of the health worker.

> The health worker was very serious. *"This is the thing that almost made me quit. Feelings! Trying to sort them out. Trying not to say the wrong thing and trying to do the right thing. Half the time I didn't know what was right or wrong. Sometimes, it seems that the more you know, the less you do. . . . Oh, blast it all, I don't know what I am saying. . . ."*

> The author was serious also. *"Learning to understand feelings, yours and your patients', will never be easy and learning how to manage your own feelings and how to make them useful tools in patient care will be a lifelong task. Are you sure you want to go on with this? You can still quit you know. There are many things you could do which would be easier."*

*The health worker made a face. "You know I am hooked
or you wouldn't say that. If I quit now, I will always
wonder what I had missed. . . ."*
*The author smiled at him. "Well then, I think we are ready
for the next principle."*

objectivity

Objectivity seems such an innocent word, but it is loaded with
all kinds of complications. Quite frequently a health worker
will find himself deeply involved in a situation in which he has
no business whatsoever. Extracting himself does not always
prove to be easy. The ability to be able to look at a situation, to
walk around it and view it from all sides before taking action
sometimes requires considerable self-discipline and experience.

If the health worker has had any opportunity to work on
research projects he will know the importance of assembling
factual data before making a judgment. Even a research-
oriented health worker, however, can forget objectivity when
confronted with human problems which arouse emotions such
as love, pity, or anger. We have already discussed cases of
abused children. An entire staff may be caught up in feelings of
horror and outrage when a badly injured child is brought into
the emergency room. If it is suspected that the parents are
responsible, it is very difficult not to show one's feelings of
anger and revulsion in dealing with them. Not only is this
reaction true of the health worker, but the police, representa-
tives of social agencies, anyone who in any way is involved in
the case may get swept up in emotions. Two things must be
emphasized in such cases. *First,* the facts may not be known. Is
one or both of the parents mentally retarded or mentally ill and
therefore not accountable for their behavior? Is one or both of
the parents so damaged by the manner in which they themselves were brought up that it can be questioned whether it is
they or the society which failed to protect them when they
were young that is the offender? Decisions such as these are
exceedingly complex and often not ones for the health worker

to make. His role is to aid in caring for the injured child. He can observe and listen, and at all times his manner must be objective.

The *second* reason for maintaining objectivity in such cases as that of the abused child is that unless the staff can remain objective, the parents may react to the anger and hostility they sense, and remove the child from care. Until a court can take appropriate legal steps, the parents can remove the child. Sometimes when this kind of thing happens, the family disappears, and no more is heard from them until the child is brought in again to some other emergency room— dead or dying from new injuries.

Such cases as these put a severe emotional strain on all the staff who work on them. It will be helpful if the health worker has someone—a supervisor, perhaps—with whom he can talk out his feelings. Putting them into words will relieve some of the tension.

Often on the geriatric ward or in a nursing home an elderly patient is seemingly neglected by his family. In some instances he appears to have been mistreated—starved or beaten. It's easy to judge the family—to assume they are responsible. Maybe they are. The health worker, however, must again remember he may not have all the facts. Even though all indications point to neglect, it is not his place or his responsibility to decide who was right and who was wrong. He has a patient who needs his care. Perhaps the patient's family needs some kindness and warmth too. Family relationships are always complicated and while no one condones or approves neglect or mistreatment, who can know all that created such a state of affairs? The patient is brought to the health care facility's attention at a moment of crisis—a severe illness, emotional, physical, or a combination of both. A crisis is never a time to make an evaluation of a family relationship. Sometimes, the true story may never be known. But the health worker must remain nonjudgmental. Objectivity does not mean coldness or withholding of concern and caring for the patient and his family. It means noninvolvement in all things not related to care of the patient.

The health worker agreed. "It means, don't try to play God with the patients or their families. It means, keep your nose clean. This, though, is another principle which sounds easier than it is. If you aren't careful, you can easily say or do the wrong thing. One thing especially can undo you. You may be doing pretty well in keeping your cool as far as the family or the patient is concerned until you notice that some of the rest of the staff don't have their feelings under control. You watch them say and do things you are certain they shouldn't do—then you have a fight with yourself to be objective about the behavior of the staff. Sometimes controlling your feelings about the staff is harder than managing your feelings about the patient and his family."

"Yes," the author agreed. "However, your feelings and attitudes toward the other staff members are as important as those toward the patient and his family. They are a part of health care."

protection

This principle, protection of the patient, means not only guarding him from harming himself or others if he is not in a responsible state of mind but also shielding him from curious people and sometimes from well-meaning friends or family. An example of this is a patient who is ordinarily extremely correct in his speech and his behavior. As part of his illness he is restless and keeps tossing the bedclothes aside, exposing himself. His language is quite colorful and, to his horrified family, vulgar and profane. The family struggles to keep him properly covered and scolds him for talking as he does. This patient needs protection from his family, unless someone can help them understand that these things are merely a part of the illness and, hopefully, when he recovers he will have no memory of them. Although the health worker may not deal directly with the family, his "unflappable" manner may be more reassuring to them than words would be.

Protection of the patient from the carelessness or thoughtlessness of the health worker or his coworkers is an equally important aspect of this principle and one not always identified.

"Right," the health worker said. "This is like the first principle—easy to overlook and to forget."

"Perhaps you can think of an example to illustrate this one," the author said thoughtfully.

"An example!" the health worker frowned as he considered this. "There was Mr. Chavez, but—maybe Mr. Ziegler would do better. Remember him? He was that old man with that fluffy white hair—baby hair we called it—who was always wandering into the wrong room. Whenever he did, whoever was in the room, a patient or a health worker, would yell, 'Wrong room, Charlie,' and he would stand there with a silly grin on his face until someone took him by the arm and said, 'Come on, you don't belong in here.' Some days it seemed as if everyone was yelling at the old man. It almost became a kind of game.

"I remember one day I took a medical chart down to the social worker's office. I didn't know until I turned around, but Charlie had followed me down there. I waited for the social worker to throw him out, but she didn't. She just smiled and said, 'Sit down, Mr. Ziegler, and visit with me for a while.' And the old man eased himself into a chair near the door and looked so pleased and kind of relieved. After that, he spent quite a lot of time in the social worker's office. She didn't seem to give him much attention, but she let him sit there and she always spoke kindly to him. While she went on about her business, he would watch the people come and go, never seemed to say anything, but acted real interested in everything that went on, although I don't think he understood very much."

"How did the other staff and the patients treat him after that?" the author asked.

The health worker looked surprised. "I don't remember. I don't think he was much of a problem after that—maybe because he had someplace where he could go and be around people—and not be yelled at. Maybe the social worker talked to some of the others . . . I really don't know. . . ."

"Whatever the reason, the patient was less upset. This is really an example of not one but two principles—acceptance as well as protection. You will find there is frequent overlap of these. The important thing is that they are recognized and applied."

The health worker nodded.

"Now tell me, do you think these six principles cover the major elements in patient care?"

The health worker thought the question over. "For the time being, yes. With more experience I may think of other things, but right now I'll have all I can do to keep these in mind and work on them. It shakes me up, you know. If I had known all this was part of caring for patients, I don't know if I would have been brave enough to tackle it. No wonder that some of the people who work in health care places are edgy and kind of hard to get along with and I include myself among them."

"Perhaps it might be helpful if you gave some thought to the skills required to apply these principles. . . ."

"What are they?"

skills utilized in application of principles

In Chapter 4 some of these elements were mentioned as means of learning more about patients. In this chapter let us think of them as skills to be acquired, to be learned and expanded as far as and in as much depth as the health worker desires. The first one to be discussed is observation.

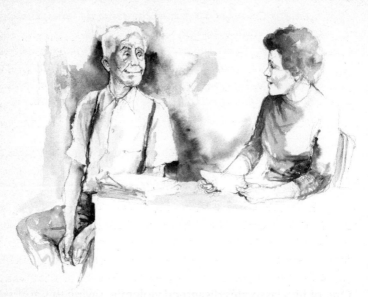

FIGURE 8
"She just smiled and said, 'Sit down, Mr. Ziegler,
and visit with me for a while.' And the old man eased himself
into a chair near the door and
looked so pleased and kind of relieved."

observation

Observation is a skill usually taken for granted. Everyone observes—if he has sight—but how can his behavior be developed and made into a valuable aid in relating to people? To use
the hunter as an example, as he walks through the woods he is
primarily interested in the trails of the animals he is hunting.
He sees marks on the trees which tell him where deer have
been feeding. A heavy clump of underbrush suggests a possible shelter for rabbits. Snow to him means only that it is
easier to identify the tracks of the creatures he wants to kill.
The more experienced he becomes, the more he is able to
identify all the signs and signals of animal habitation. Unless he

is an unusual person, he is unaware of the beauty of the landscape, the patterns made by the branches of the trees, the color and texture of the leaves, the birds and their songs. All these things mean little to him unless they relate in some way to hunting. Much observing is like looking down a long tunnel and seeing only those things directly in front of it. Many people do this—see only the end but not the things along the way.

How can observation, effective observation, be learned? One psychology student thought he had an answer. He had to walk through the business section of the city on his way to and from work and while walking he made a mental inventory of the objects he observed in the show windows. Once he arrived at his office or home, he wrote down all the things he could remember. He said that each day his list grew longer and that this exercise helped him sharpen his powers of observation. One of his classmates disagreed violently, saying this approach was not a valid experiment.

How stupid to fill one's mind with a clutter of utterly useless objects. I am a people watcher. As I walk down a street, attend a football game, go any place where there are crowds of people, I pick out individuals and try to see how much I can learn about them, their moods, their occupations, the kind of people they are. The only trouble with this kind of observation is that you are not sure how accurate your observations are. However, when I apply such a method to the patients I work with, I can check my impressions. I try to see how much I can learn about them before I talk with them. I watch their interaction with other patients or staff. I notice their dress, the way they sit, how they handle their cigarettes. I try to make some guess as to their age and to the kind of problem they have. I do all observing and predicting before I have read their chart or the referral slip. If later in my interview I find I have been reasonably accurate in my impressions, I feel like Sherlock Holmes. When I miss what later seems obvious, I try to think back to my initial observations and see what misled me. I have come to feel that such practice is a very useful exercise in learning about people.

A staff sergeant in World War II tells of a base surgeon he knew.

The surgeon used to say that he could make a fairly accurate estimate of the morale of his company from his ward rounds each day. And he could. Sometimes it was difficult to know how he did it. I never felt I really knew. He would walk around with a little notebook, make a few marks in it now and then, go through all the wards, the mess hall, the clinic, surgery—stopping now and then to have a few words with one of the staff or a patient. Then he would return to his office, sit down at his desk, take out his notebook, write a few memos, and maybe call in one or two of the staff for a conference. I don't think he missed a thing, from the thickness of the potato peelings in the mess hall to the private in the storeroom who had received a "Dear John" letter the day before and had been drinking too much since then. It seemed like magic sometimes, how he knew some of the things he did. He called it trained observation!

No one will know how many times in health care facilities poor or inaccurate observation has led to mistakes in diagnosis and treatment. In most institutions little formal training exists for such aspects of health care as observation. Here again, the health worker will find he must devise his own ways of self-training.

evaluation

Hand-in-hand with observation is the skill of evaluation. So closely are they related that it is difficult to discuss one without discussing the other. Just to observe an incident is not enough. One must interpret the incident or decide what it means. For example, the health worker sees a patient crying. It is not enough merely to observe the patient crying. He must determine what the tears mean. Are they tears of anger, fear, pain, loneliness, or depression? Far too often most people, not just health workers, jump from observation to action based on some quick assumption, ignoring the in-between step of evaluation. In the example of the crying patient, tears may mean a much-needed release of tension and the action indicated may be no action except to protect him from the interference or curiosity of others.

"Hey, wait just a minute," the health worker said in great alarm. "This is getting too deep for me. How will I know if my evaluation is right? How will I know what to do if it is?"

"To evaluate is a more difficult and subtle skill than to observe and make a neat little list of all the things you have seen. But you are doing more evaluation than you realize. You are doing it all the time. What I am trying to do is make you aware of how important and useful a tool evaluation can be.

"Think about a mother with her child. She learns the meaning of her baby's cry—whether it indicates hunger, anger, or a wet diaper. She didn't learn this out of a book. She learned it out of close and loving association with her baby.

"The base surgeon didn't start out a 'trained observer.' He started out, just as you, by observing the things around him. Then, just as you, he began to wonder, to question, and to try to evaluate the significance of what he saw. He too made mistakes, many of them at first. Only after much experience did he become an expert.

"Let's look at another example:

"A psychiatrist was teaching a class of students from the schools of nursing, social work, and psychology. He described the case of a mentally ill person, by describing behavior and the symptoms. Quoting from the medical record, he repeated some of the things the patient had said. He then asked the class what the diagnosis was.

There was silence and then one of the nursing students said timidly, 'We aren't supposed to make a diagnosis.' The psychiatrist snorted. 'I am not asking you to write a diagnosis on the chart, but how in heaven's name can you know what to say, what to do, or when to call a patient to my attention unless you can make an 'educated guess' as to the diagnosis?

"*The psychiatrist continued, 'That's all a diagnosis is to a physician, an educated guess, subject to change when he gets new information. It's only a guideline to be considered as such, a signpost, the cap on a bottle. Among yourselves or in your own minds I know you have some ideas about the diagnosis. I am asking you to tell me what they are. If you are wrong, I will tell you. But don't just sit there.'*"

The author stopped. Then she went on, "*You do this kind of practical evaluation all the time. You observe. You evaluate what you observe. Let us take an example. You are walking down the hall and you see a patient in a wheelchair who appears to have come from the emergency room. One of your coworkers is wheeling him toward the elevator. Now what does that scene suggest to you?*"

The health worker answered slowly. "*Well, I would think that here is a patient who came to the emergency room, was examined there, and is now being admitted to the hospital.*" *He hesitated and then went on speaking slowly,* "*I would wonder what was wrong with him. If he showed any scratches or bruises I might think he had been in an accident. If he were very sick he would more likely have been on a stretcher. He could be coming in for minor surgery or a routine checkup. Sure, I would wonder what was wrong with him, but I wouldn't have much to go on. It could be so many different things.*"

"*But you would be not only observing but trying to evaluate what you saw. Conscious evaluation is what I am trying to teach you to do. What else would you look for?*"

"I'd try to guess how old he was. And I would try to see if I could tell how he was feeling. I would look for any sign he was in pain."

"That is the kind of thing I am trying to teach you—to observe, to evaluate—even when viewing a situation we have been talking about."

The health worker was not satisfied. *"How am I going to know if my evaluation is right?"*

"How would you test it?"

The health worker was thoughtful. He frowned a little. *"Well,"* he said slowly, *"I would probably know the attendant who was taking him up to the ward and I could make it a point to ask him about the patient, which ward he was taking him to, what he knew about the patient— not where the patient could hear me"* he said hastily, *"but sometime later. Or, I know most of the people in the ER and I could talk with some of them, maybe look at the chart if it hadn't already been sent upstairs. . . ."* The health worker stopped and frowned more deeply. *"I don't know about doing all of that though. It doesn't feel right somehow. . . . Well, blast it all."* He stopped and got up and began pacing the floor.

"Go on," the author said quietly, sitting still and erect and watching him closely.

"Well," he said getting up from his chair and pacing the floor. Finally, he turned toward the author. Pointing his finger at her accusingly, he continued, *"It would be a kind of snooping, wouldn't it?"*

The author relaxed and permitted herself a slight smile. *"It would. It's what we call an invasion of privacy, isn't it? And even though it's important that you learn how to observe and to test your evaluations you cannot do so at the expense of a patient, can you? Now it's possible that our hypothetical patient might be assigned to you for some service, and within the limits of that service you would be able to check your observations, but you should not go beyond those limits. For example, you might be asked to get a blood sample. In the process of establishing rapport with the patient you could find out what he does and where he came from. You could also try to determine something of how he is feeling and make a guess as to his preliminary diagnosis, but you should not probe into matters which are personal and private."*

The health worker looked relieved. "I get you. Curiosity about a patient is one of those areas where a lot of health workers make mistakes. They don't mean to. Mostly, they are interested but sometimes it turns out to look like nose trouble."

listening

Few people listen. A history professor comments on this:

I am reasonably conscientious. I try to prepare a good lecture, but I know only a handful of students will listen to it. Some of the students will read newspapers while I speak, some just sit in some sort of stupor, locked in an inner world of their own. Sometimes I have an impulse to turn handsprings in order to get their attention. . . .

A nurse said:

I remember. I shall always remember the old man who years ago cried out in deep anguish to me. "You don't understand what I am trying to say! Can't you listen? Can't you listen?" It wasn't until years later that I understood what he was trying to tell me. Then I was young, inexperienced, preoccupied with my own affairs, concerned only with showing everyone how efficient, how brilliant I was. How cruel we can be to the people we think we are helping.

A young woman who had a fractured leg and wore a cast for several weeks talked of her experiences:

You know, I was surprised. People would come up to me, often complete strangers, and ask how I had broken my leg, and then before I could tell them, they would interrupt to tell me of their broken leg or of someone they knew who had had one. I had the feeling everyone in the county had had a broken leg at one time or another. I was fascinated about how few people were interested in what had happened to me. Not that it was all that unusual, but . . .

How many times a patient is asked, "How do you feel today?" And how often he answers, "Just fine." Both question and answer have become a ritual without much meaning. Students in health care facilities will say, "But we don't have time to listen to all the things the patients want to talk about." How do you get students to understand that intelligent listening may *save* time and help to more correctly assess a patient's real condition? Years ago in social work, the students were required to write out or dictate verbatim the interviews they had with their clients. Then the supervisor would go over the interviews with the students asking such questions as, "Why do you think the client said that? What do you think he meant by that expression? What would have happened if you had not interrupted?" It was a painful way of learning the importance of listening.

Once the health worker accepts the fact that listening, intelligent listening, is important, that, in itself, is an important step in mastering the listening skill. Evaluation is closely related to good listening, also. The health worker must frequently ask himself, "Was that what the patient really meant? Why did he say that? Did I make the proper response?" Often the answer to this last question will be "no" until he has considerable experience.

The health worker squirmed in his chair. "Listening is one skill that bugs me. I always think, too late, 'You should have kept your big mouth shut, you fool.' I get caught up in all the things there are to do, but I guess that isn't a good excuse, is it, the being-too-busy bit?"

"No. It isn't, but you are not the only one who uses it. Keep trying. Listening gets easier with practice."

communication

Most of the skills discussed in this chapter relate to communication. The word "communication" is so overworked and so often abused and misused that it is difficult to find new and original things to say about the subject. Scientists say that animals and insects have a highly developed communication system. Human communication, in spite of all that has been said and written about it, is still imperfect. Someone will say, "I don't think we are communicating," and another person will say, "My vibes tell me you don't like me." Patients in a group therapy class were asked to give examples of good communication. One patient said she thought her husband was very skillful in communicating.

> *He knows what to say and how to say it in such a manner that it gives me great support and encouragement when I need it most. But he also knows when to remain silent and just gather me in his arms and hold me till my fears go away.*
> *"If you have all that going for you, I don't see what you are doing here," a second patient said enviously.*
> *"I did not always appreciate what I had," the first patient replied quietly. "I just took it without question. . . ."*

Communication includes both sending and receiving. It means observing nonverbal cues, interpreting signals, listening, and responding both verbally and nonverbally. As the body-language interpreters point out, we often communicate without realizing it.

Touch is an important element in nonverbal communication. One therapist, wise woman that she is, makes it a point to embrace her clients when they arrive at or leave her office because she knows that troubled people often feel alone and isolated from their own kind. Used inappropriately this kind of action would not be wise. Dying patients often find great comfort in having someone hold their hand. Words do not seem to help them as much. Patients going into surgery respond gratefully to a reassuring pat on the shoulder. Some of the group sensitivity training sessions make quite a point of touching as one means of communicating.

Recently three small children arrived from France to visit their grandparents. They spoke no English, but communication was never a problem for them. Their small, vivid faces were alight with interest and enthusiasm and they raced from one new experience to another, laughing and chattering, their arms outstretched as if to embrace the whole world. Everyone was charmed by them. There was a father who said, "My daughter never met a stranger."

Such incidents suggest that perhaps we try too hard to communicate. Instead of "acting naturally" we make communication a project. Communication should be as natural a process as breathing, but we labor over it. We hold classes, write books, arrange formulas.

"You mean," the health worker said, "if we took a deep breath and relaxed, the communication thing would fall into place, the right words would come out, the right things would be done?"

The author shook her head. "I don't mean we oversimplify. Communication is too important a part of our relations with others. It does take work—hard work—but I think sometimes we overshoot our target because we are so deadly serious. It is also well to keep in mind that the way one communicates is a very personal thing and you will find that beyond a certain point there can be no imitation. You must walk alone. . . ." "No," she said in response to the puzzled look on the health worker's face," I am not going to explain that. I want you to think about it. . . ."

action

"To do the right thing at the right time and in the right way" is a skill that needs to be viewed with caution. "Do something. Don't just stand there," is the thought that goads us into activity—sometimes useless or even harmful activity.

The health worker has ample opportunity for action in the

performance of his regular duties. However, in interaction with patients, their families, or other staff members he must consider a different kind of behavior and sometimes nonaction is required.

For example, after surgery, patients are often required to cough and deep-breathe in order to keep their lungs clear. Most patients comply although many do not understand the reason for this coughing and breathing. Sometimes, though, the health worker may discover a patient who is only half-heartedly doing the exercises. His first impulse is likely to be a "let's-have-no-nonsense" attitude and to attempt to *make* the patient breathe properly. However, he should proceed cautiously. First, he might want to be sure he knows how to do the exercises. Then, depending on the patient and the relationship he has with him, the health worker might probe very gently to learn why the patient resists this procedure. "You don't like doing this, do you?" he may say. Often the patient may give the health worker a reason for his reluctance to cooperate. A common one is that he has known of someone who had a rupture or hemorrhage after surgery and died. Whatever the reason, the health worker must handle it seriously and kindly, but usually any explanation of why the procedure is necessary should be left to the professional. He may say calmly, "Lots of patients worry about these exercises. I guess we didn't explain them to you. I am going to have the nurse come in and answer some of your questions." The health worker's matter-of-fact acceptance of the patient's fears can be very reassuring. Yet his activity was limited to identifying the problem and seeing that it was reported to the proper source for action.

The health worker sighed. "Action, as a skill, is a hard one. I'll just have to keep working on it though."

"You have been given a lot of hard-to-digest material in this chapter."

"Well, I asked for it, but it's enough to keep me busy for a while. Relations with people, interaction, understanding, respect, this whole bit of caring for people is full of

dynamite. Do, don't do, listen, think . . ." he stopped and shook his head.

"But?" the author queried.

"Oh, I like it. When you begin to understand the things we've been talking about here, even if you only half get them it adds a lot to your job."

"New dimensions?" the author asked.

"I guess you could call it that. . . ."

SUMMARY: In this chapter the health worker has been given what he asked for: some guidelines. They should be considered only that. Any list of principles of human behavior can be dangerous if they are considered the only means of relating to people, the only way to help and care for people, particularly the sick. These principles are intended merely to help the health worker increase his understanding and to encourage him to go on learning.

The health worker will see there is considerable overlap among these principles. How can you, for example, have awareness, concern, and objectivity without having respect for people? Can any of these principles be applied if the capacity to feel for and with people is not present?

The skills mentioned here suggest some of the ways the principles can be applied but are intentionally not described in detail. In any learning experience in the behavioral sciences true learning begins only when the student begins to rearrange the ideas he is receiving and puts in concepts born out of his own experience and understanding—inputs which will change as he continues to learn.

ASSIGNMENT: Your assignment for this chapter is a longer one than usual:

1 Take the following table and under each of the principles check the skills you think should be used to apply them. For your reassurance, there is no right or wrong list. Today you may check them in one way. Tomorrow,

PRINCIPLES

SKILLS	Respect	Awareness	Acceptance	Concern	Objectivity	Protection
Observation						
Evaluation						
Listening						
Communication Verbal						
Communication Nonverbal						
Action						

events will occur which will lead you to check them in another way. This kind of change sometimes is called professional growth.

2 Look at the skills listed in the chart on page 248. Think about them for a little while and then write down at least one way you can apply each of them.

conclusion

This book was designed and written for a special audience—the health worker. In spite of having responsibility for 90 percent of patient care, the health worker has been poorly equipped to understand the emotional needs of patients or to recognize his own feelings about illness and to appreciate how they affect his ability to care for patients. Seldom, if ever, is the health worker's role defined except in terms of technical competence. Yet, there has never been a greater need to identify and treat the human needs of patients and health workers than in today's health care programs. Implied in the narratives found in this book and conversations with health workers and patients throughout the health care system is the plea for small, intimate signals that they, health worker and patient alike, have some identity as persons and that they be valued and respected.

Unfortunately, modern technological advances in the health field have hindered rather than encouraged a personalized approach to patient care. This should not be. There can be a fusion between the objectivity of the scientist and the humanistic approach. There must be a union of this fusion if the patient is to have the best of medical and surgical procedures and at the same time retain his personal identity and some semblance of self-respect and well-being. However, a marriage between two such separate elements of patient care will never be successful until as much money, as much time, as much recognition of the importance of the "human element" is granted as is now given to the technological or scientific aspects of patient care.

The humanistic or "caring" part of the health worker's responsibilities has been the emphasis of this book. Here, as in any book on human relations, there are methods or ideas which will be challenged. Dissent, however, often has its positives, because it is out of differences that new concepts may be born. It is not important that the health worker accept or reject the ideas he has read in this book. It is important that from it he gain an awareness of the value of patients as people, and that he be motivated to continue to learn about the things that are of concern to people when they are sick, and how he, as a health worker, can best help them. Only when he has learned successful interaction with people can he achieve his full potential as a health worker.

The author and the health worker stood looking at the manuscript ready for mailing to the publisher.

"Our book is finished," the author says with deep satisfaction.

"Do you think anyone will read it?" the health worker asks worriedly.

"Of course," she says, speaking with more assurance than she feels.

"I hope so," says the health worker, eyeing the manuscript with a paternal kind of pride. "But," he added, "you know what? I'm going to miss our arguments."

"There's one very good solution for that. We'll start another book."

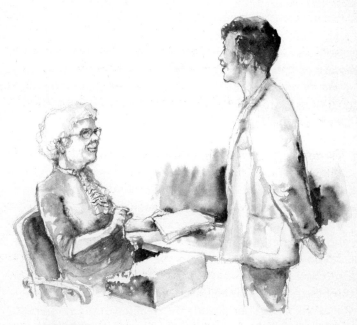

FIGURE 9
"Our book is finished," the author says with deep satisfaction.

bibliography

This bibliography does not and could not include all the books and magazines which would be useful to the health worker. As he seeks to extend his knowledge and understanding of the health field, of patients, and of himself, the health worker will find that a part of the satisfaction in learning comes from the search and discovery of material which first arouses his interest and then leads into the development of new awareness and new ways of handling his daily tasks.

The health worker will be fortunate if his institution offers seminars or institutes which he may attend, but in addition to that kind of education he should locate the nearest library and learn the art of browsing into strange books and magazines and, as he can afford it, begin to collect some of the books which he finds most useful. Many of the books he will use now come in paperback. For a small fee libraries will provide copies of special chapters or articles from magazines.

The health worker should learn to use a medical dictionary and the reference section in the library. A book on the introduction to medicine such as the textbook used by freshman medical students may be useful. He will need to know some of the popular nontechnical magazines in the health field as well as the more specialized. The health worker's supervisor or other staff members may suggest special articles or books, but if he truly wishes to learn he will take the initiative in seeking new knowledge. The following list suggests some areas for the health worker to explore:

magazines

Family Health. Family Health Magazine, Inc. 1271 Avenue of the Americas, New York, N.Y. 10020.

Hospital and Community Psychiatry. American Psychiatric Assn. 1700 18th St., N.W., Washington, D.C. 20009.

Hospital Physician. Medical Economics, Inc., 550 Kinder-Kamack Rd., Oradell, New Jersey 07649.

Hospitals. Journal American Hospital Assn. 540 N. Lakeshore Drive, Chicago, Ill. 60610.

Psychology Today. Communications Research Machines. Carmel Valley Road, Del Mar, Calif. 92014.

Today's Health, American Medical Assn. 535 N. Dearborn St. Chicago, Ill. 60610.

(Other more technical journals and magazines will be found in county medical society libraries, medical school libraries, and in some of the libraries of larger institutions.)

reference books

Adams, F. Dennette, M.D.:*Physical Diagnosis,* 14th ed., Williams and Wilkins Co., Baltimore, 1958.

Blakiston's Pocket Medical Dictionary, 3d ed., McGraw-Hill Book Co., New York, 1973.

magazine and newspaper articles and pamphlets

Anonymous: "Children's Ward," *The Atlantic,* vol. 191, no. 2, pp. 34–37, February 1953.

"Caring Is Part of the Cure," *The Johns Hopkins Magazine,* pp. 1–17, Spring 1971.

Hudson, Charles L., M.D.: "Whatever Became of That Old-fashioned Patient?," *The Journal of the American Medical Association,* vol. 203, no. 8, pp. 143–145, Feb. 19, 1968.

Lang, Priscilla A. and Oppenheimer, Jeanette R.: "The Influence of Social Work When Parents Are Faced with the

Fatal Illness of a Child," *Social Casework,* vol. 49, no. 3, pp. 161–166, March 1968.

Loeser, Katinka: "Whose Little Girl Are You?," *The New Yorker,* vol. 38, no. 20, July 7, 1962.

Mosher, Lawrence: "When There Is No Hope: Why Prolong Life?," *The National Observer,* vol. 11, no. 10, p. 1, Mar. 4, 1972.

Shepherd, Jack: "Black Lab Power," *Saturday Review,* vol. 55, no. 32, pp. 33–39, Aug. 5, 1972.

Statement on a patient's bill of rights. American Hospital Association, Lakeshore Drive, Chicago, Ill., 1972.

"Your Rights as a Patient at Beth Israel Hospital Boston," Beth Israel Hospital, 330 Brookline Ave., Boston, Mass., 02215.

books

Anderson, Kenneth E.: *Introduction to Communication Theory and Practice,* Cummings Pub. Co., Menlo Park, Calif., 1972.

Bernstein, Lewis and Richard H. Dana: *Interviewing and the Health Professions,* Appleton-Century-Crofts, New York, 1970.

Bloom, Samuel W.: *The Doctor and His Patients,* The Free Press, New York, 1965.

Burling, Temple, M.D., Edith M. Lentz, Ph.D., Robert N. Wilson, Ph.D.: *The Give and Take in Hospitals: A Study of Human Organization in Hospitals,* G. P. Putnam's Sons, New York, 1956.

Crichton, Michael: *Five Patients: The Hospital Explained,* Alfred A. Knopf, New York, 1970.

Curtin, Sharon: *Nobody Ever Died of Old Age,* Atlantic Monthly Press Books; Little, Brown, Boston, 1973.

Duff, Raymond S., M.D., and August B. Hollingshead, Ph.D.: *Sickness and Society,* Harper & Row, New York, 1968.

Editors of Fortune: *Our Ailing Medical System,* Perennial Library; Harper & Row, New York, 1969.

Hays, Joyce Samhammer, B.S., M.S., R.N., and Kenneth H.

Larson, B.S., R.N.: *Interacting with Patients*, Macmillan Co., New York, 1963.

Kübler-Ross, Elisabeth: *On Death and Dying*, The Macmillan Co., New York, 1969.

Reik, Theodor: *Listening with the Third Ear*, Arena Books, Pyramid Publications, Inc., New York, 1972.

Somers, Anne R.: *Health Care in Transition: Directions for the Future*, Hospital Research and Education Trust, Chicago, 1971.

Steiger, William and A. Victor Hansen: *Patients Who Trouble You*, Little, Brown, Boston, 1964.

Sussman, Marvin B. et al,: *The Walking Patient: A Study in Outpatient Care*, Cleveland Press of Case Western Reserve Univ., 1967.

Taylor, Carol: *In Horizontal Orbit: Hospitals and the Cult of Efficiency*, Holt, Rinehart, and Winston, New York, 1970.

Wheelis, Allen: *The Quest for Identity*, W. W. Norton & Company, Inc. New York, 1958.

Wolcott, Lester E., M.D. and Paul C. Wheeler, M.D.: *Working with Older People. Vol. IV, Clinical Aspects of Aging*, Public Health Service Publication No. 1459, July 1971, U.S. Dept. of Health, Education and Welfare, Public Health Service, Rockville, Md. 20852.

Zborowdki, Mark: *People in Pain*, Jossey-Bass Inc., San Francisco, 1969.

index